STUDY GUIDE TO ACCO

HUMAN INTIMACY

MARRIAGE, THE FAMILY AND ITS MEANING

SEVENTH EDITION

FRANK COX
Santa Barbara City College

PREPARED BY
MARY ELIZABETH STIVERS, PH.D.
Middle Tennessee State University

DUANE STUCKY, PH.D.
Middle Tennessee State University

WEST PUBLISHING COMPANY
Minneapolis/St. Paul   New York   Los Angeles   San Francisco

WEST'S COMMITMENT TO THE ENVIRONMENT

In 1906, West Publishing Company began recycling materials left over from the production of books. This began a tradition of efficient and responsible use of resources. Today, 100% of our legal bound volumes are printed on acid-free, recycled paper consisting of 50% new paper pulp and 50% paper that has undergone a de-inking process. We also use vegetable-based inks to print all of our books. West recycles nearly 27,700,000 pounds of scrap paper annually—the equivalent of 229,300 trees. Since the 1960s, West has devised ways to capture and recycle waste inks, solvents, oils, and vapors created in the printing process. We also recycle plastics of all kinds, wood, glass, corrugated cardboard, and batteries, and have eliminated the use of polystyrene book packaging. We at West are proud of the longevity and the scope of our commitment to the environment.

West pocket parts and advance sheets are printed on recyclable paper and can be collected and recycled with newspapers. Staples do not have to be removed. Bound volumes can be recycled after removing the cover.

Production, Prepress, Printing and Binding by West Publishing Company.

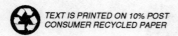

TEXT IS PRINTED ON 10% POST CONSUMER RECYCLED PAPER

Printed with **Printwise**
Environmentally Advanced Water Washable Ink

ISBN 0–314–08975–6

Contents

Preface

Welcome to the *Study Guide to Accompany Human Intimacy: Marriage, The Family, and Its Meaning* by Frank Cox. In this study guide, you will find helpful summaries, questions, and answers to assist you in fully covering and learning the important material in the text by Frank Cox. The intention here is twofold: to help you review and study the text by yourself, and to provide questions to answer and discuss that will not only assist your individual study but will help you study in a group. Our goal is to help you learn the material as well as developing your critical thinking and analytical skills.

This study guide augments each chapter of the text in five ways:

Chapter Outline: An outline of the important facts and issues is provided. Blanks have been provided in the outline so you can interactively review the text and the outline together.

True-False Questions: Questions are provided to probe your understanding of the material.

Key Terms: In each chapter, the most important terms for you to remember are covered in the fill-in-the-blank section.

Multiple-Choice Questions: Twenty-five questions are provided for each chapter.

Critical Thinking and Decision Making: Several questions are provided to assist you in clarifying your own opinions about issues, to help you look at all factors associated with issues, and to provide discussion material with other individuals.

In several chapters, special discussion questions are provided for *Examining International Families*. In the respective chapters, the author reviews the characteristics of families in other cultures. The questions will help you compare the American culture to others.

Chapter 1
Making Decisions That Lead To Successful Relationships

Chapter Outline

Prologue: Strengths of Successful Relationships
- _____ means experiencing intense, intellectual, emotional, and physical communion with another human being.
- Without intimacy, there is emotional isolation which increases the risk of physical and emotional disorders.
- The family in which we were born and grew up, our family of _____ , is the first seat of all of our learning, and human relationships are the essence of the family.

Qualities of Strong and Resilient Families: An Overview
- Vera and David Mace coined the phrase "_____" to describe the strong family that is functioning successfully.
- Mace(s) and Stokol maintained that healthy families help to develop healthy community environments. The quality of life in families is in turn strongly affected by the quality of relationships between couples who founded those families.
- Six qualities shared by strong, healthy families are: _____ , _____ , good communication patterns, desire to spend time together, a strong value system, and the ability to deal with crises and stress in a positive manner.

Making Decisions That Lead to a Fulfilling Life

- Human beings have the longest dependency period of any mammal. A long socialization period is necessary to learn how to adapt successfully to society and to make the decisions that lead to a satisfying life.
- Successful _____ develops high self-esteem, the capability of understanding and relating positively to others, and the ability to make good decisions that lead to a fulfilling and productive life.

Logic and Emotion in Decision Making

- When we make decisions without knowing or being aware of the decisions, they are made _____ . When we are aware and know we have made a decision, we have made the decision _____ .
- A successful decision strikes a balance between both the rational and emotional aspects of a given situation.

Decision-Making Steps

- The six general steps of decision-making are:
    1. _____ .
            Set and order of priorities.
            Consider both short- and long-term outcomes.
            Differentiate between logic and truth.
    2. _____ .
            Seek advice from others.
            Approach decisions in a systematic manner.
    3. _____ .
            Sort out relevant influences.
            Use common sense and intuition.
            Avoid stereotypical thinking.
            Avoid confusion between words and their meanings.
            Avoid mistaking correlation for causation.
    4. Identify, evaluate, and compare your choices.
            Use numerical weighting.
            Set minimum standards.
            Consider the negatives.
    5. Make your decision, develop a plan, and get started.
            Avoid snap decisions.
    6. Evaluate your decision and readjust it if necessary.
            Stay flexible.

Theoretical Approaches to Family Study
- _____ focuses on social structures and organizations and the relationships between them.
- _____ focuses on interactions between individuals.
- Three different theoretical perspectives are:
  The _____ approach which tends to concentrate on institutions such as family, school, church, or government.
  _____ which views the world in terms of conflict and change and tends to produce a critical picture of society with an emphasis on social activism and criticism.
  _____ theory which focuses on how individuals interact and examines the subjective personal meanings of human acts.

Can We Study Intimacy?
- Family science is the study of marriage and family.
- It is within the family that most of us learn to be intimate, caring, loving people. Thus, the study of family is also the study of intimacy.

Some Words About Marriage and Family Data
- Most data on families come from surveys, from clinicians who work in the field, and from direct observations of families.
- Surveys are problematic for three reasons:
  1. _____ .
  2. _____ .
  3. It is difficult to validate respondent's answers.
- _____ data are usually anecdotal and conclusions may be over-generalized. Group data do not accurately predict what an individual will do.
- _____ is difficult to arrange, and the presence of the observer modifies the family's behavior.

Family and Nation: Government Family Policy
- Houlgate suggests six legal functions that concern families:
  1. _____ : laws that impose fines to ensure compliance.
  2. _____ : laws that define particular grievances and specific remedies.
  3. _____ : laws that are designed to protect specific persons, usually children, from harm.
  4. Conferring private power: laws that give private persons legal power.
  5. Conferring public power: laws that give public persons, such as courts, legal power.
  6. Benefit/burden distribution: laws that provide cash assistance, housing, and employment.

African American, Latino, and Asian American Families

- The principle of _____ states that people are attracted to others who share similar objective characteristics such as race, religion, ethnic group, education, and social class.
- _____ make up the largest minority in the US. The most important economic change in the last 40 years for African Americans has been the emergence of the middle class, partly because of higher educational attainment.
- Latino families comprise about _____ percent of the US population. More recent immigrants have less schooling and less English language ability and therefore are less able to find economic success. Those who have been in the US for a long period of time are economically more successful.
- Asian American comprise about _____ percent of the US population. On the whole, they are better educated, occupy higher occupational positions, and earn more that the general US population.

Summary

- Research suggests six major qualities of strong, healthy families: commitment to the family, appreciation of family members, good communication skills, the desire to spend time together, a strong value system, and the ability to deal with crises and stress in a positive manner.
- Learning to make good decisions and choices is important to the creation of strong and successful intimate relationships and families.
- Research on relationships, marriage, and the family is guided by a variety of theoretical perspectives including structural functionalism, conflict theory, and symbolic interactionism.
- Research on relationships, marriage, and the family is more prone to subjective bias.
- Social institutions, especially governmental bodies, greatly influence the family as well as individual Americans.
- American society is made up of a great diversity of peoples.

Key Terms

1. When one experiences intense intellectual, emotional, and when appropriate, physical communion with another person it is referred to as being _____.
2. The family in which one is born into is called _____.
3. Focusing on the relationships between social structures and organizations is called

   _____.
4. The study of interactions between individuals is called _____.
5. "Likes tend to marry likes" illustrates the principle of _____.
6. A _____ is an inflexible, fixed belief about something that may be only partially correct.
7. Individuals make hundreds of decisions every day, some of which are made _____ and some _____.

True-False Questions

1. _____ Having a vision of what we want for ourselves, our relationships, families, children, society, and the world is of the utmost importance to human beings.
2. _____ Stinnett and DeFrain's research suggests that rigid religious doctrines that promote only traditional sex roles or negative approaches to family planning might be detrimental to family life.
3. _____ A successful decision is one that strikes a balance between both the rational and emotional aspects of a given situation.
4. _____ When trying to make good decisions, it isn't important to distinguish between the logic of an argument and the truth behind the logic.
5. _____ A correlation between two things determines the cause.
6. _____ The inability to identify choices is one of the major characteristics of troubled people.
7. _____ In the field of family studies, most data comes from direct observations.
8. _____ Most family laws are criminal in nature.
9. _____ Individuals need to decide on the theory they think best explains intimate relationships and utilize that theory when trying to understand all behavior.
10. _____ One characteristic of a strong family is the desire to spend time together.

Multiple-Choice Questions

1. Family wellness refers to
   a. a family that is on the road to recovery after a crisis
   b. a strong family that is functioning successfully
   c. a family that is physically healthy
   d. a community support system

2. Of the six major qualities shared by all strong families, which is the most important?
   a. appreciation
   b. good communication patterns
   c. commitment
   d. strong value system

3. Which quality of a strong family is most often expressed as a high degree of religious orientation?
   a. a strong value system
   b. ability to deal with crisis in a positive manner
   c. commitment
   d. appreciation

4. Organized religion may be advantageous to family life by
    a. sponsoring family activities
    b. enhancing the family's support network
    c. providing social and welfare services
    d. all of the above

5. Which is not one of the characteristics that successful socialization develops?
    a. an outgoing personality
    b. high self-esteem
    c. the capability of understanding and relating positively to others
    d. the ability to make good decisions

6. An immediate understanding of something without conscious reasoning or thinking is called
    a. common sense
    b. preconceived idea
    c. intuition
    d. connotative

7. Which of the following statements is true about correlation and causation?
    a. a correlation determines causation
    b. do not infer causation from mere correlation
    c. the two are totally unrelated
    d. none of the above are true

8. The family theory that identifies social structures and examines how they function is called
    a. exchange theory
    b. conflict theory
    c. symbolic interaction
    d. structural-functional theory

9. The family theory that tends to produce a critical picture of society with emphasis on social activism is called
    a. symbolic-interaction
    b. conflict theory
    c. structural-functional
    d. role theory

10. The family theory that examines the subjective personal meanings of human acts is called
    a. symbolic-interaction theory
    b. conflict theory
    c. structural-functional
    d. exchange theory

11. What percentage of people marry at least once in their life time?
    a. 98%
    b. 75%
    c. 90%
    d. 80%

12. Which is not one of the problems associated with survey research?
    a. it is difficult to validate respondents' answers
    b. self-report data reflects their opinion
    c. anonymity cannot be guaranteed
    d. the sample may not be representative of the population being studied

13. Which is not one of the three types of data collection used in the family field?
    a. survey data
    b. clinical data
    c. direct observation
    d. rating scales

14. Which type of data collection is the hardest to conduct?
    a. clinical data
    b. survey data
    c. direct observation
    d. anecdotal records

15. Which type of data is the hardest to generalize to a larger population?
    a. survey data
    b. clinical data
    c. direct observation
    d. experimental research

16. Laws that impose fines or use imprisonment to ensure compliance are called
    a. penal
    b. regulatory
    c. remedial
    d. burden distribution

17. Statutes that make parents liable for at least a limited amount of damage to other's property caused by children's vandalism is called
    a. regulatory
    b. conferring public power
    c. penal
    d. remedial

18. Child custody laws are an example of which type of laws?
    a. benefit/burden distribution
    b. conferring private power
    c. conferring public power
    d. regulatory

19. Which statement accurately represents Danziger and Gottschalk's research on the effects of welfare on family stability?
    a. state welfare programs destabilize families
    b. welfare policies have no real dramatic effect on family structure
    c. welfare programs create family stability
    d. none of the above

20. Which of the following statements is true about African American families and income?
    a. the income disparity between Caucasian married couples and African American married couples has greatly decreased over the past decade
    b. African American family income has increased very little in the past decade
    c. lower class African American family's income has experienced the greatest percentage growth compared to other minorities
    d. the income disparity between Caucasian married couples and African American married couples has greatly increased over the past decade

21. Who is the largest minority in the United States?
    a. Latinos
    b. Asian Americans
    c. Indians
    d. African Americans

22. Asian Americans are often perceived as a "model minority" because they
    a. occupy higher occupational positions
    b. are better educated
    c. earn more than the general US population
    d. all of the above

23. Which is not one of the major qualities of a strong family?
    a. commitment
    b. sense of humor
    c. good communication patterns
    d. appreciation

24. An idea or opinion that one holds before knowing all the facts is called
    a. a stereotype
    b. a connotative opinion
    c. a preconceived idea
    d. intuition

25. Which minority may constitute a higher percentage of the population than the census figures indicate due to illegal immigration?
    a. Latino
    b. Asian American
    c. African American
    d. European Americans

Critical Thinking and Decision Making
1. Compare and contrast the three theories of family interaction.
2. Would you consider your family to be a strong family? Why or Why not?
3. How would you rate your family on the six major qualities of a strong family?
4. Up to this point in your life, overall, do you think you have made good decisions? Why or Why not?
5. Choose a bad decision that you have made in your life and analyze it using the six steps of decision making. Where did you falter?

Examining International Families
1. Discuss the pros and cons of having the government control the family as opposed to the family governing itself.
2. Are there similarities between the governments of the US and Canada regarding their role in the family?

Answers

Key Terms: 1   intimate
              2   family of origin
              3   macrosociology
              4   microsociology
              5   homogamy
              6   stereotype
              7   consciously, unconsciously

True/False: 1 T; 2 T; 3 T; 4 F; 5 F; 6 T; 7 F; 8 F; 9 F; 10 T

Multiple Choice: 1 b; 2 c; 3 a; 4 d; 5 a; 6 c; 7 b; 8 d; 9 b; 10 a; 11 c; 12 c; 13 d; 14 c; 15 b; 16 a; 17 d; 18 c; 19 b; 20 a; 21 d; 22 d; 23 b; 24 c; 25 a

Chapter 2
Human Intimacy, The Family and Its Meaning

Chapter Outline

- An assumption is a belief that may or may not be supported by facts.
- Modern families seem to have shifted from being child centered to being adult centered.

<u>Family: The Basic Unit of Human Organization</u>
- Assumption 1:
    The _____ is the basic unit of human organization. If defined functionally, it is essentially universal. However, its structural form and strength may vary greatly across cultures and time.
- Broad definition of family: the system society uses to support and control reproduction and sexual interaction.
- Narrower definitions of family:
    <u>Census Bureau:</u> two or more persons related by birth, marriage, or adoption and residing together. Households are defined as all persons occupying a housing unit.
    <u>Sociologist (Gere):</u> a structure that carries out childrearing and is characterized by kinship.
    <u>NY Court of Appeals:</u> "It is the totality of the relationship as evidenced by dedication, caring and self-sacrifice of the partners."
    <u>National Opinion Poll:</u> Over 70 percent included married couples with or without children, a divorced parent living with her/his children, a never-married parent living with her/his children, and an unmarried couple who have lived together for a long time and are raising children.
    <u>Beutler:</u> A family must include ties across generations established by the birth process.
- Confusion exists because alternate forms are being used to carry out the functions of a family.

Family Functions

- The family serves society as well as the individual:

    _____ .

    _____ .

    Provisions must be made to resolve conflicts and maintain order.

    Children must be socialized into society.

    Intimacy, emotional gratification, dealing with emotional crisis, and developing a sense of purpose are harmonized with societal values.

- The contemporary American family fully serves only two of society's needs: _____ and

    _____ .

Sexual Regulation

- Unlike other animals, humans can seek and enjoy sex at any time. In most societies, the family is the basic institution for controlling sexual expression in a manner that meets the needs of the society as a whole.

- _____ : Having many sexual partners.

- _____ : Having multiple spouses.

- _____ : Having one spouse in a sexually exclusive relationship.

- Each culture establishes a "correct" system of sexual control.

- The family's function has changed over time and will continue to change. However, it is likely that the need for primary affection bonds, intimacy, economic subsistence, socialization of the young, and reproduction will continue to be handled through the family structure.

The American Family: Many Structures and Much Change

- Assumption 2:

    A free and creative society offers many structural forms by which family functions, such as childrearing, can be fulfilled.

- Family structure: the parts of a family and their relationship to one another.

- Stereotypically, two parents and children are a _____ family.

- The single-parent family has been one of the fastest growing family structures with the proportion of children living with one parent growing from 12 percent to 30 percent from 1970 to 1993.

- The increase in single-parent families is largely due to the high divorce rate, but to a lesser, growing extent, the greater acceptance of the unwed mother has also contributed to the increase.

- When a nuclear family becomes a single parent family, e.g. through divorce, and the single parent remarries, the family becomes a _____ family.

- Available alternatives for intimacy have increased. Family patterns and gender roles are less stereotyped and rigid. Cohabitation has become a relatively permanent family structure. Singlehood and marriage without children have gained more acceptance.

- America's acceptance of changing family patterns is mainly economic and partly philosophic. Affluence from industrialization and greater educational/ career opportunities for women make it possible to consider alternate lifestyles and marital forms.
- Having broader choices of acceptable relationships means that intimate relationships are generally less stable. The more choices available, the more the chances that mistakes may be made.
- Former structures restricted the possibilities for self-growth and social contributions; current structures require improved understanding of the consequences of decision-making to enjoy more fully the opportunities available.

Change Within the Continuity and Uniqueness Within Commonality
- Assumption 3:
    Family life involves continuity as well as change.
- Assumption 4:
    Each family is unique but also has characteristics in common with all other families in a given culture.
- Change can occur within continuity. Uniqueness can exist within commonality.
- Family permanence has continued at about the same level for the past century. In 1900, the majority of marriages ended with the death of one of the spouses. Today, about one divorce occurs for every two marriages compared to one for every twelve in 1900. However, divorced persons still return to the institution of marriage.
- The falling birthrate does not mean that fewer women are opting to have children. Families are producing fewer children on the average which is probably positive for children, but families are still having and rearing children.
- The proportion of single-parent families remained at about _____ in ten from 1870 to 1970. Early single-parent families resulted from death rather than divorce as is true today.
- Recent changes in family life appear deviant only when compared to the 1940s and 1950s. In the broader picture of social change, today's young people appear to be behaving in ways consistent with long-term historical trends.
- During the 1920s, common-law cohabitation involved one in five couples. Today, there are still only 6 unmarried couples per 100 married couples.
- Statistics on cohabitation include, for example, young persons living with an elderly person for economic reasons. One should be wary in interpreting the statistics to mean that young people are rejecting marriage.

Family: A Buffer Against Mental and Physical Illness
- Assumption 5:
    The family becomes increasingly important to its members as social stability decreases and people feel more isolated and alienated. Indeed, the healthy family can act as a buffer against mental and physical illnesses.

- Empirical studies suggest that _____ persons generally appear happier and less stressed than _____. It becomes a matter of health then to work toward improved family functioning and increased levels of intimacy.
- A healthy family can act as a buffer against mental and physical illnesses of its members. An unsuccessful family may do the opposite.

The Need for Intimacy

- _____, _____, and _____ closeness to others seem to be basic needs of most people. It is within the family, that such feelings ideally are most easily found and shared.
- Intimacy: experiencing the essence of one's self in intense intellectual, physical and/or emotional communion with another human being.
- The primary components of intimacy are choice, mutuality, reciprocity, trust, and delight.
- Intimacy is a process, not a state of being. It can be considered on what three dimensions:

    _____

    _____

    _____

- As economic patterns have changed and geographic mobility has increased, social emphasis has shifted from family closeness to individual fulfillment. Individuals have found _____ more difficult to achieve.
- Couples must seek carefully a satisfactory mix of intimacy inside and outside the marriage.
- List the four barriers to intimacy:

    _____

    _____

    _____

    _____

The Family as Interpreter of Society

- Assumption 6:

    The attitudes and reactions of family members toward environmental influences are more important to the socialization of family members than are the environmental influences themselves.

- _____ : internalizing society's rules, mores, taboos, etc.
- The family is the main avenue for socializing preschool children. Formal education takes on part of the job later.
- Sociopaths or psychopaths: persons with inadequate conscience development, irresponsible or impulsive behavior, inability to maintain good interpersonal relationships, rejection of authority, and inability to profit from experience.
- _____ : learning by observing other peoples' behavior.
- Parents and other family members are the most significant models for young children, and their reaction to social changes will teach their children values. Thus, attitudes toward racial prejudice, tolerance, law, and authority are established.

- If the family shares the general society's values, it will help its children become responsible community members. Thus, strengthening families strengthens the community itself.

Unique Characteristics of the American Family
- Assumption 7:
    The American family, especially the middle-class families, has certain characteristics that make it unique. Among these, the following stand out:

    _____

    _____

    _____

    _____

Family: The Consuming Unit of the American Economy
- Assumption 8:
    The family is the basic economic unit in modern America.
- Money earned by outside work supports the family. The family buys what it needs and becomes the basic consuming unit of society.
- The health of the economy depends on consumer spending. Thus, the family acts as an economic foundation of American society.

Family: A Resilient Institution
- Our image of families in the past is often based on myth rather than reality. Aging wasn't a problem because people died before they got old. Adolescence wasn't a difficult stage because children worked and education was a privilege of the rich.
- Families have changed from formal, authoritarian, rigidly disciplined institutions with rigid sex roles to patterns characterized by interpersonal relationships, mutual affection, sympathetic understanding and comradeship.
- The family can easily adapt to the new emphasis on personal and relational growth and development.
- We need to expend more energy on making marriage and family viable and fulfilling than on suggesting alternatives to them.

Strengthening the Family
- In the national debate to strengthen the family, two extremes stand out as agenda for change. They are:

    _____

    _____

- Returning the structure to the 1950s would require reversing the move for greater opportunities for women and for improving economic conditions of the family.

- Extensive government programs to subsidize families, especially "non-nuclear" ones, seems to be successful when viewing European welfare states. Thus, it seems inevitable that the United States will move in this direction. However, the movement would weaken the family.
- There is a third alternative. We could seek to invigorate the family within the changed circumstances of our time. We should stress that the "me" attitude has gone too far and reinvigorate the sense of community.
- The supreme importance of families to a strong society should be recognized, and ways should be suggested for families to adapt to modern conditions of individualism, equality, and gender equality.
- The family institution is flexible and resilient, and it can adapt to modern changes. A strong, healthy family is the individual's greatest source of love and intimacy.

Summary
- Human intimacy is based on eight assumptions about marriage and the family in America:
    1. The family is the basic unit of human organization.
    2. A free and creative society offers many structural forms by which family functions, such as childrearing, can be fulfilled.
    3. Family life involves continuity as well as change.
    4. Each family is unique but also has characteristics in common with all other families in a given culture.
    5. The family becomes increasingly important to its members as social stability decreases and people feel more isolated and alienated.
    6. The attitudes and reactions of family members toward environmental influences are more important to the socialization of family members than are the environmental influences themselves.
    7. The American family, especially the middle-class family, has certain characteristics that make it unique.

Key Terms
1. A belief that may or may not be supported by the facts is called a(n) _____.
2. The basic unit of society is considered by many to be the _____.
3. According to the US census bureau, all persons who reside in a single family dwelling are referred to as a

   _____.
4. Being in a _____ relationship means a person has only one spouse.
5. A _____ has two or more spouses.
6. People who have multiple sexual partners are often referred to as being

   _____.
7. The author defines the _____ family as a married couple and their children who reside together.
8. When a parent remarries, this family is referred to as a _____ family.

9. _____ is when one or both spouses have sexual partners outside the marriage and each partner accepts the arrangement.

10. Each family is _____ yet families also _____ over time as well as maintain _____.

11. A feeling of emotional and intellectual closeness within a family is referred to as _____.

12. The five components of intimacy are _____, _____, _____, _____, and _____.

13. Biddle suggests that the three dimensions of intimacy are _____, _____, and _____.

14. Supplying skills for functioning in society is referred to as _____.

15. People who cannot function in society are referred to as _____.

16. Learning through observation of others is called _____.

True-False Questions

1. _____ The major difference between families and other relationships is the permanence of the relationship.

2. _____ Single parent families are transitional family forms.

3. _____ Today, young people have broader choices of acceptable relationships which has made intimate relationships more stable.

4. _____ The birthrate has decreased over the years mainly because women are choosing careers over children.

5. _____ Research indicates that children do better in smaller families because they receive more parental attention.

6. _____ Over ninety percent of men and women will marry at least once in their lifetime.

7. _____ Families have become more of a refuge for its members who have been bruised and battered in the outside world.

8. _____ To love and be loved is a basic need of most individuals.

9. _____ Self-disclosure does not lead to deeper levels of interaction because most people become turned off by what they see in others.

10. _____ Because society has shifted from family closeness to individual fulfillment, people have found intimacy more difficult to achieve.

11. _____ Over time, a strong network of friends is the most helpful toward individual fulfillment and happiness.

Multiple-Choice Questions

1. The most important change that has occurred in families today is
    a. new individual freedoms for women
    b. the shift from child centeredness to adult centeredness
    c. the increase of various family forms
    d. the shift from adult centeredness to child centeredness

2. Which of the following is not a necessary function of the family?
    a. replacement of dying members
    b. techniques for solving conflicts and maintaining order in the family
    c. socialization of children
    d. provision for leisure activities

3. Having multiple spouses is referred to as
    a. polygamy
    b. promiscuity
    c. monogamy
    d. polyandry

4. When two or more nuclear families share a common spouse, this is referred to as a
    a. tribal family
    b. concubine
    c. composite family
    d. commune

5. The turmoil of the 1960s and 1970s made many contributions to society, the most important was
    a. less stereotypic gender roles
    b. an increase in available alternatives for intimacy
    c. freedom not to marry
    d. none of the above

6. All but one of the following changes has helped women become more independent and less dependent on marriage, it is
    a. more women in the labor force
    b. increased education for women
    c. increase in the minimum wage
    d. the women's movement

7. Until 1970, single parent families were created mainly through
    a. divorce
    b. desertion
    c. adoption
    d. death

8. Coombs' review of recent research indicates that _____ persons tend to be happier and less stressed.
    a. married
    b. divorced and separated
    c. widowed
    d. single

9. When partners give to the relationship and to each other, it is called
    a. delight
    b. trust
    c. openness
    d. reciprocity

10. The dimension of intimacy that refers to the sharing of meaningful self-disclosures is called
    a. breadth
    b. depth
    c. openness
    d. none of the above

11. The belief that each individual must find deep intimacy to become a self-actualized and fulfilled person is espoused by
    a. Freud
    b. Maslow
    c. Biddle
    d. Kieffer

12. Which is not one of the strongest barriers to intimacy?
    a. expressed anger
    b. fear of rejection
    c. unexpressed anger
    d. nonacceptance of ourselves

13. Which of the following is the main avenue for socializing children to American culture
    a. schools
    b. family
    c. peer group
    d. television

14. Middle-class American families have certain characteristics that make them unique. Which of the
    following is not one of those characteristics?
    a. freedom in mate and vocational selection
    b. high economic standards and abundant personal possessions
    c. relative freedom within the family
    d. extreme openness of families

15. One of the following is not a way that the author addresses to deal with problems facing families today
    a. return to the structure of the traditional family of the 1950's
    b. develop extensive government policies to help families
    c. place more stringent regulations on all media forms
    d. reinvigorate the spirit of community

16. Richard Geles defines a family as
    a. all persons who occupy a housing unit
    b. a group of two or more persons related by birth, marriage, or adoption and residing together
    c. persons who support each other emotionally and financially
    d. a social group and institution that possesses structure and carries out specialized functions

17. In a national opinion poll, less than half of the respondents listed one of the following as a family
    a. never married mother living with children
    b. two lesbians who are raising children
    c. a cohabiting couple
    d. a married couple with no children

18. The American family has full responsibility for only two of the primary functions; they are
    a. supplying human replacements and providing emotional gratification and intimacy
    b. socialization of children and providing emotional gratification and intimacy
    c. solving conflicts and establishing individual goals
    d. solving conflicts and replacing dying members

19. Which of the following has been one of the fastest growing family forms during the past decade?
    a. married couples without children
    b. never married singles
    c. single parent families
    d. married couples with children

20. Compared to the past, modern America is
    a. less tolerant of multiple forms of intimate relationships
    b. more tolerant of multiple forms of intimate relationships
    c. more accepting of multiple forms of intimate relationships
    d. as accepting of multiple forms of intimate relationships

21. Which of the following statements is true about cohabitation?
    a. the number of young couples who live together in a sexually and emotionally intimate relationship
       has increased steadily
    b. the data are unclear because we really don't know what happens within these relationships
    c. cohabitation has decreased over the past twenty years
    d. none of the above

22. The dimension of intimacy that refers to the sharing of true, central, and meaningful aspects of
    themselves is referred to as
    a. depth
    b. breadth
    c. openness
    d. trust

23. Which is not a characteristic of a sociopath?
    a. inability to maintain good interpersonal relationships
    b. irresponsible behavior
    c. rejection of authority
    d. development of a conscience

24. Families are often blamed for the problems of their individual members? Families are also influenced by
    a. unemployment
    b. economic depression
    c. civil unrest
    d. all of the above

25. Since 1970, the number of women living alone has increased
    a. 50 percent
    b. 75 percent
    c. 90 percent
    d. 40 percent

Critical Thinking and Decision Making

1. Are American families really fulfilling their major functions in order to maintain society? Why or why not?
2. Will families be non-existent in thirty years? Why?
3. How does affluence affect people lives?
4. What things in your life, if any, would you change if you suddenly acquired $100,000?
5. Do youth of today accept responsibility for their actions or do they expect someone such as parents to get them out of trouble?

Debate the Issues

Should society allow persons of the same sex to marry? Why or why not?

Answers

Key Terms:
1. assumption
2. family
3. household
4. monogamous
5. polygamist
6. promiscuous
7. nuclear
8. reconstituted or blended
9. swinging
10. unique; change; continuity
11. intimacy
12. choice, mutuality, reciprocity, trust, delight
13. breadth, openness, depth
14. socialization
15. sociopaths
16. modeling

True/False: 1 T; 2 T; 3 F; 4 F; 5 T; 6 T; 7 T; 8 T; 9 F; 10 T; 11 F

Multiple Choice: 1 b; 2 d; 3 a; 4 c; 5 b; 6 c; 7 d; 8 a; 9 d; 10 c; 11 b; 12 a; 13 b; 14 d; 15 c; 16 d; 17 b; 18 a; 19 c; 20 b; 21 b; 22 a; 23 d; 24 d; 25c

Chapter 3
American Ways of Love

Chapter Outline

- American culture believes that love should be the basis for marriage.
- Courtly love, which began among feudal aristocracy, glorified love from afar and made a fetish of suffering over love affairs. Marriage love was considered unexciting and mundane.
- Ancient Japan regarded love as a grave offense if not properly sanctioned, for it interfered with arranged marriages.
- Today, 87 percent of various cultures throughout the world recognize romantic love.
- Today, India still places responsibility for finding a mate on the parents or older relatives.

The American Myth That Romantic Love Should Always Lead to Marriage

- Crosby suggests that the American idea that romantic love should lead to marriage is a myth. Therefore, numerous marriages have little more than love going for them and dissolve because the couple has no other basis to build a lasting relationship.
- Love does play a role in marriage, and even in arranged marriages, couples often build a loving relationship over time.
- Love has many meanings and does not take just one form.

Defining Love

- The Greeks divided love into a number of elements, three of which are:

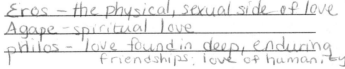

  Eros – the physical, sexual side of love
  Agape – spiritual love
  philos – love found in deep, enduring friendships; love of humanity

- The _philos_ element of love is most important in giving society its humanity.
- The family primarily teaches moral values that foster philos love.

Theories of Love
- Various theories of love have little empirical support.
- Fromm suggests:
    Brotherly love: _is characterized by friendship & companionship w/ affection_
    Maternal love: _is characterized by an unselfish interest in your partner._
- Fromm includes four basic elements in mature love in addition to sexual response: _care_, _responsibility_, _respect_, and _knowledge_.
- Casler suggests that love develops, in part, because of our need for acceptance and confirmation. We tend to attach ourselves to someone who offers validation. The validation may be more a product of dating, i.e. developed over time, as opposed to an innate attraction.
- Society emphasizes the necessity for love to precede sex. Thus, some persons fall in love quickly to avoid the frustration or anxiety of waiting for sex.
- Reiss suggests four stages in a wheel as a model for love:
    Stage 1 _Rapport_: partners become comfortable with each other and want to deepen the relationship.
    Stage 2 _self-revelation_: partners share intimate thoughts and feelings and self-disclose.
        Women are more likely to reveal their thoughts and feelings. Self-revelation is higher among couples having egalitarian attitudes toward gender roles.
    Stage 3: _mutual dependent_: partners feel at a loss if the other is not present.
    Stage 4: _personal need fulfillment_: needs commonly concern intimacy.
    Our sociocultural background and role conceptions influence how quickly we move through the stages.
- Goldstine suggests three stages:
    Stage 1 _falling in love_: both partners are excited and see the good points and ignore the bad points.
    Stage 2 _disappointment_: shortcomings are recognized and couples learn to accept them.
    Stage 3 _acceptance_: confidence and trust help bring the relationship into balance.
- Sternberg suggests three elements within love: _intimacy_, _passion_, and _commitment_. He then identifies types of love in terms of the three elements:
    Nonlove: absence of all three elements
    Liking: intimacy only
    Infatuation: passion only
    Romantic love: intimacy and passion without commitment
    Companionate love: intimacy and commitment without passion
    Fatuous (foolish) love: passion and commitment without intimacy
    Empty love: commitment without passion and intimacy
    Consummate love: intimacy, passion, and commitment together
- Numerous theories exist. All describe love as having many parts and/or developing through stages.

Romantic Love

- Romantic love is an idealized image characterized by "love at first sight", "the one and only", and the "perfect mate". It is only a set of attitudes about love.
- Often, persons mask qualities in others that do not fit their idealized image. They fall in love with their romantic ideas rather than their partners.
- Confusion between romance and love causes difficulty in forming long-lasting intimate relationships.
- Romance alone does not recognize and accept the reality of differences and shortcomings of partners. Dating and broad premarital experience can help correct romantic idealism.
- As emotional, intellectual, social, and physical intimacy develops, romance becomes one of several aspects of a relationship, not the only one.

Infatuation

- Some say romantic love and infatuation are the same thing. The difference may be only semantic. Infatuation is used to negate past feelings of love that have now changed.
- Others suggest that infatuation is the first step toward love. Infatuation is less mature and permanent than love.
- Love is learned, and part of learning to move toward a mature, realistic love may be simply trial and error.
- The most important prerequisite for true love may be knowing and accepting ourselves.

Loving and Liking

- One can love someone you dislike, but the dislike will probably lead to the breakdown of the relationship.
- Liking each other is probably more important than loving each other in successfully living together for an extended period of time.
- Hendrick and Hendrick suggest that liking and loving are the same and all that differs is the persons' interpretation of the situation.
- + reinforcement and + associations are important in maintaining a "like" relationship.
- Davis suggests that friendship includes the following essential characteristics: enjoyment, acceptance, trust, respect, mutual assistance, confiding, understanding, and spontaneity. He further suggests that love relationships also include the characteristics of a Passion cluster (fascination, exclusiveness, and sexual desire) and a Caring cluster (giving the utmost and being a champion/advocate).

Love Is What You Make It

- Each person defines love in a unique way for them from life experiences. Therefore, couples must agree on what love and acts of love are, and must act on their agreement to maintain love in their relationship.

- Fehr surveyed a number of people to determine their description of the central features of love (in order):
  - trust
  - caring
  - honesty
  - Friendship
  - Respect
  - Concern for the other's well-being
  - Loyalty
  - Commitment
  - Acceptance of way the other person is
  - Supportiveness
  - Wanting to be with the other
  - Interest in the other
- Strong physical attraction, emotional attachment, and a feeling of openness are also generally important in loving relationships.
- The Principle of Least Interest: the indifferent person, who cares least in a relationsh. exercises more control over relationship. The other person is more vulnerable and is eager to placate and please.
- Personal growth and venturing into new feelings or unknown areas of oneself are also part of the love experience.
- Because love is uniquely defined by each individual, often partners may not perceive when love is expressed to each other. Women's concepts of love are emotional expressiveness, intimate sharing, discussing the relationship, and saying "I love you", while men tend to show their love in more practical ways such as being a good family provider.
- Love is what you make of it through your attitudes and behaviors.

Love in Strong Families: Appreciation and Respect

- Mature love always includes appreciation of the loved ones. Strong families seem to start a circular process: I appreciate and respect you, you learn to appreciate and respect yourself, which leads you to appreciate and respect me.
- A vicious circle is a pattern of behavior in which negative behavior provokes a negative reaction, which in turn prompts more negative behavior.
- Respect is an important quality of strong families.
- Constructive criticism: criticism given in a manner, attitude, and tone that will promote improvement and development.
- Appreciation includes respect for privacy. Everything about every family member need not be shared with all members of the family. Each family member may need time alone.
- Members of strong families are able to receive appreciation gracefully. Inability to accept appreciation stifles further expressions of appreciation.

Styles of Loving

- Lasswell and Lobsenz believe love can be classified in six general styles:

  best friends: comfortable intimacy from close association over a period of time, seldom with the assumption of developing into love or marriage

  game playing: a challenge or contest in which intimacy is encouraged but held at arm's length

  logical: pragmatic search for the kind of partner with which a permanent relationship can be developed; relationships last as long as they are perceived as a fair exchange.

  possessive: consumed by the desire to possess the beloved totally and to be possessed by the lover

  romantic: the love of love experience itself and the image of passion, intimacy, and intensity

  unselfish: unconditional caring and nurturing, giving and forgiving, and even self-sacrificing

Learning to Love

- The meaning of love and how to demonstrate it is learned from those around us: siblings, parents, peers, and from the general culture in which we are raised. Thus, how we express and define love is the result of our past experiences.

Actions and Attitudes

- Conflicting attitudes and unrealistic expectations arise from differing past experiences and cause difficulties in developing interpersonal relationships.
- Attitudes consist of three components:

  Affective: due to one's emotional response

  Cognitive: due to beliefs or factual knowledge

  behavioral: how one acts as a result of an attitude
- Socialization: the learning and development of basic attitudes from other members of society
- Children pass through various stages of development as they grow to adulthood.
- Freud delineated four psychosexual stages leading to adult sexual and love expression:

  Self-love Stage (infancy and early childhood):
  Almost all energy is focused on oneself and exploring the environment.

  Parental Identification stage (early and middle childhood):
  The roles associated with gender are developed.

  Gang Stage (late childhood and preadolescence):
  Each gender tends to avoid the other. Consolidation of appropriate gender role and cooperation are developed.

  Heterosexual Adult stage (onset of puberty and after):
  All that is learned in previous stages plays a role in developing a map of what love is, how it is displayed, and suggesting characteristics of the person to be loved.

Love Over Time: From Passionate to Companionate Love

- Murstein defines companionate love as a strong bond including tender attachment, enjoyment of the other's company, and friendship.
- Romantic love tends to become companionate love in an enduring relationship.
- Compare romantic love and companionate love:
    Romantic love: thrives on <u>deprivation, frustration, high arousal level, & absence</u>.
    Companionate love: thrives on <u>contact & requires time to develop & mature</u>.
- When children arrive, a couple's love broadens to include them and a greater portion of the love is agape love or selfless love. If love continues to develop, it will become a mixture of romantic, selfless, and companionate love.
    May describes this mixture as <u>authentic</u> love.
    Fromm describes this mixture as <u>mature</u> love.
- In authentic or mature love, giving takes precedence over taking. Partners develop a reciprocal relationship in which giving and accepting reinforces one another.
- Love continues to change throughout a lifetime as social, physical, intellectual, and emotional aspects change.
- American culture presents obstacles to an enduring relationship by exalting aspects of passionate or romantic love. Consequently, many Americans equate sex with love. Our culture also emphasizes the individual which leads to preoccupation with oneself, self-improvement, and self-actualization.
- Baker suggests that the importance of sex should be de-emphasized and that sex should flow spontaneously from a relationship filled with love, joy, struggle, growth, and intimacy.
- Etzioni suggests that marriage is often less an emotional bonding than a <u>breakable alliance</u> between two self-seeking individuals.
- Passionate love tends to preclude all but oneself and the beloved. Thus, there would be no sense of community in society if only passionate love existed. Companionate and passionate love will find a healthy balance in an enduring relationship.
- Clearly, thought and work are required to remain in love.

Love's Oft-Found Companion: Jealousy

- Jealousy may be defined as the state of being resentfully suspicious of a loved one's behavior toward a suspected rival. It derives from feelings of insecurity and inferiority.
- Envy is <u>a discontent w/ oneself and/or a desire for the possessions & attributes of another</u>
- Jealousy is characterized by a sense of feeling lonely, betrayed, afraid, uncertain, and suspicious. Envy elicits shame, longing, guilt, denial, and a sense of inferiority.
- Jealousy is related somewhat to the rules our culture teaches. Behaviors that my instill jealousy in one culture may not in another culture.
- In American culture, love has meant exclusivity. Therefore, every interaction of a partner with the opposite sex provides an opportunity for jealousy to arise.

- Characteristics of American jealousy:
  - Jealousy goes with feelings of insecurity and an unflattering self-image.
  - Jealousy is often derived from one's own unfaithfulness.
  - Jealousy occurs more often in those who are more dissatisfied with their lives.
  - Desire for exclusivity is the strongest predictor of jealousy.
  - Younger people are more often jealous than older people.
  - Women suffer more from jealousy than men.
  - Women try to repair the damaged relationship, whereas men try to repair their damaged egos.
  - Jealousy is a problem in one-third of relationships.
  - Men are more apt to break up over a women's infidelity than the reverse.
  - Women are more apt to try to induce jealousy in men than the reverse.
- As American sexual mores have loosened, the need for jealousy has diminished.
- Hansen found that nontraditional sex role subjects were less jealous than traditional sex role subjects.
- Steps to manage and control jealousy:
  We can try to learn what is making us jealous.
  We can try to keep our jealous feeling in perspective.
  We can negotiate w/our partners to change certain behaviors that trigger jealousy.
  Choosing partners who are reassuring & loving will also help reduce our irrational jealousies.

Summary
- American youths are given relative freedom to choose a mate.
- Love is difficult to define.
- Our attitudes and personal definition of love lead us to form a set of idealized expectations as to the kind of mate we desire.
- Attitudes about love and marriage develop through a number of stages as one grows from infancy to adulthood.
- The stages of development are only theoretical constructs and vary with culture and individuals.
- It is important to like as well as love our mate if a relationship is to endure.
- Jealousy is an oft-found, yet unwanted companion of love.

Key Terms
1. Love that is altruistic, giving, and nondemanding is called __agape__.
2. Love that is found in deep and enduring friendships is referred to as __philos__.
3. Needing, desiring, and wanting another person physically is called __eros__ love.
4. __Brotherly__ love is characterized by friendship and companionship with affection.
5. When an individual places a partner's needs ahead of their own, that person is demonstrating __Maternal__ love.

6. According to Erich Fromm, the four basic elements necessary in any intimate relationship are _Care_, _Responsibility_, _Respect_, and _Knowledge_.

7. In Reiss' theory of love, the _Rapport_ stage is when partners are comfortable with each other and both want to deepen the relationship.

8. In the _Self-revelation_ stage of Reiss' theory of love, the partners want to deepen the relationship through self-disclosure.

9. As sharing becomes more and more intimate, feelings of _mutual dependency_ develop in Reiss' theory of love.

10. As partners deepen their relationship, they experience _personal need fulfilment_ which leads to the establishment of more rapport.

11. Goldstine believes that love occurs in three stages; they are _falling in love_, _disappointment_ and _acceptance_.

12. According to Sternberg, the absence of all three elements is referred to as _non love_.

13. Intimacy and passion without commitment is called _Romantic love_.

14. A combination of intimacy, passion, and commitment are referred to as _Consummate love_.

15. Intimacy without passion or commitment is referred to as _liking_.

16. Passion without intimacy or commitment is called _Infatuation_.

17. Passion and commitment without intimacy is called _fatuous (foolish) love_.

18. Commitment without passion and intimacy is referred to as _Empty love_.

19. Intimacy and commitment without passion is called _Companionate love_.

20. The concept of _Romantic Love_ embraces such ideas as "love at first sight" and "the one and only."

21. Romantic love in retrospect has been referred to as ~~the perfect mate~~ _infatuation_.

22. A ~~Confusion b/c romance & love~~ _Strong physical attraction_ is characterized by experiences of general emotional arousal when thinking of the loved one or being in her/his presence.

23. When physical attraction is accompanied by a(n) _emotional attachment_ there is a tendency to idealize and be preoccupied with the other person.

24. When two people feel they can confide in each other, they have established a _feeling of openess_.

25. The opposite of love is _indifference_.

26. The principle of _least interest_ states that the person who is the least interested in the relationship has the most power.

27. An expansion of self due to a love experience is referred to as _personal growth_.

28. When a mature loving relationship exists, the expression of _appreciation_ permeates the relationship.

29. When negative behavior promotes more negative behavior, this is referred to as a _vicious circle_.

30. When one person holds another person in high regard, this is referred to as _respect_.

31. Helping a person, in a positive way, to see their faults is called _constructive_.

32. Attitudes towards others consist of three components, they are _affective_, _cognitive_, and _behavioral_.

33. Sigmund Freud identified four psychosexual stages that lead to adult love expression. They are
_____Self love_____, _____Parental identification_____,
_____Same sex_____, and ____heterosexual adult____.

34. Love that includes tender attachment, enjoyment of each other, and friendship is called
_____Companionate_____.

35. _____Jealousy_____ stems from insecurity in one's self and in the relationship.

True-False Questions

1. __T__ In Reiss' theory, the four stages are really one process because need fulfillment was the original reason for feeling rapport.

2. __T__ In reviewing all the theories on love, one can surmise that love has numerous parts and/or develops through a series of stages.

3. __F__ People don't really fall in love with each other, they fall in love with love.

4. __T__ Men who hold traditional romantic ideals deny their own dependence needs and the independence needs of the woman.

5. __F__ As emotional, intellectual, social, and physical intimacy develops, romance dissipates.

6. __F__ Individuals are born with the ability to love; it cannot be learned.

7. __T__ The only real difference between liking and loving is the depth of our feelings and the degree of our involvement with the other person.

8. __T__ Love involves self-disclosure and self-disclosure involves risk.

9. __F__ Love is an intellectual concept rather than an emotional concept.

10. __F__ American men tend to show their love through emotional displays such as sex while women try to show their love by doing things for their partner.

11. __T__ It is impossible to create a widely accepted definition of love because each person creates their own definition through their own attitudes and behaviors.

12. __T__ We often treat the ones we love worse than others that we know.

13. __T__ The way we define and express love are the results of our past experiences.

14. __T__ Loving is a reciprocal relationship; we must be able to accept it, as well as give it.

Multiple-Choice Questions

1. Most Americans state that the main reason why they marry is
    a. convenience
    b. companionship
    c. love
    d. financial security

2. The most important prerequisite for true love is
    a. acceptance of our partner
    b. knowing and accepting ourselves
    c. understanding the person's strengths and weaknesses
    d. none of the above

3. The romantic myth of love states
    a. true love will conquer all
    b. there can only be one true love
    c. people are not reasonable when they fall in love
    d. love alone should determine who and when one should marry

4. Which of the following is not one of ancient Greeks forms of love?
    a. feta
    b. agape
    c. Eros
    d. philo

5. According to Erich Fromm the type of love that is unselfish is called
    a. brotherly
    b. consummate
    c. maternal
    d. none of the above

6. Reiss' theory of love and intimacy is
    a. linear
    b. circular
    c. curvilinear
    d. vertical

7. In Reiss' theory of love, when a partner is needed in order to feel complete, a person is in which stage?
    a. rapport
    b. personal need fulfillment
    c. self-revelation
    d. mutual dependence

8. In Reiss' theory of love, when two people have the feeling that they have known each other before, they are in what stage?
     a. rapport
     b. personal need fulfillment
     c. mutual dependence
     d. self-revelation

9. In Goldstine's theory of love, when couples take off the "rose-colored glasses," they are in what stage?
     a. acceptance
     b. disappointment
     c. falling in love
     d. self-revelation

10. Which of the following is not one of the elements in Sternberg's theory of love?
     a. intimacy
     b. commitment
     c. companionship
     d. passion

11. In Sternberg's theory of love, commitment without passion and intimacy is
     a. nonlove
     b. empty
     c. infatuation
     d. fatuous

12. In Sternberg's theory of love, passion without intimacy or commitment is
     a. liking
     b. romantic
     c. companionate
     d. infatuation

13. In Sternberg's theory of love, a combination of intimacy, passion, and commitment is
     a. consummate love
     b. companionate
     c. fatuous love
     d. romantic love

14. Keith Davis felt that romantic relationships would share all of the characteristics of friendship but would also have two additional characteristics, they are
   a. passion and commitment
   b. caring and understanding
   (c) passion and caring
   d. respect and commitment

15. According to Davis, friendship includes all of the following but one.
   a. enjoyment
   b. confiding
   c. understanding
   (d) advocacy

16. What reason is given most often for getting divorced?
   a. abuse
   (b) loss of love
   c. irreconcilable differences
   d. mistrust

17. The opposite of love is
   a. hate
   b. liking
   (c) indifference
   d. non of the above

18. According to Lasswell and Lobsenz, love that is the most unfulfilling and disturbing is
   (a) possessive love
   b. romantic love
   c. unselfish love
   d. game-playing love

19. According to Lasswell and Lobsenz, love that concentrates on practical values is
   a. unselfish love
   b. romantic love
   c. best friend's love
   (d) logical love

20. Attitudes generally consist of three components. Which is not one of those?
    a. affective
    b. behavioral
    c. cognitive
    d. subjective

21. In which stage of Freud's psychosexual development do children learn the masculine or feminine role?
    a. parental identification stage
    b. group or same sex-stage
    c. self-love stage
    d. heterosexual adult stage

22. In which stage of Freud's psychosexual development do individuals focus all their sexual energy and energy for love on themselves?
    a. heterosexual adult stage
    b. self-love stage
    c. group or same-sex stage
    d. parental identification stage

23. Which of the following is not one of the findings in Murstein's research on sex differences in love?
    a. men are less willing to marry without being in love
    b. in general, men appear initially more geared to romance than women
    c. men tend to fall in love earlier than women
    d. once a woman commits herself to a man, she becomes more expressive than the man

24. Which of the following is not an obstacle to an enduring love relationship?
    a. our culture's emphasis on the individual
    b. our culture's emphasis on community
    c. the equating of sex with love
    d. none of the above

25. Which of the following is not characteristic of jealousy?
    a. jealousy tends to cause men greater suffering than women
    b. jealousy goes with feelings of insecurity
    c. happy or not, jealous people feel strongly bound to their mates
    d. it is difficult to conceal jealousy from others

Critical Thinking and Decision Making
1. Compare and contrast Reiss,' Sternberg's, and Goldstine's theories of love.
2. How does one know when s/he is really in love?
3. Is jealousy ever beneficial to the relationship? Why? If yes, when?
4. Explain the difference between envy and jealousy?
5. How do you define love?

Answers

Key terms:		
	1	agape
	2	philos
	3	eros
	4	brotherly
	5	maternal
	6	care, responsibility, respect, knowledge
	7	rapport
	8	self-revelation
	9	mutual dependence
	10	personal need fulfillment
	11	falling love, disappointment, acceptance
	12	nonlove
	13	romantic love
	14	consummate love
	15	liking
	16	infatuation
	17	fatuous love
	18	empty love
	19	companionate love
	20	romantic love
	21	infatuation
	22	strong physical attraction
	23	emotional attachment
	24	feeling of openness
	25	indifference
	26	least interest
	27	personal growth
	28	appreciation
	29	vicious circle
	30	respect
	31	constructive
	32	affective, cognitive, behavioral
	33	self-love, parental identification, same sex, heterosexual adult
	34	companionate
	35	jealousy

Answers (cont'd)
True/False: 1 T; 2 T; 3 F; 4 T; 5 F; 6 F; 7 T; 8 T; 9 F; 10 F; 11 T; 12 T; 13 T; 14 T

Multiple Choice: 1 c; 2 b; 3 d; 4 a; 5 c; 6 b; 7 d; 8 a; 9 b; 10 c; 11 b; 12 d; 13 a; 14 c; 15 d; 16 b; 17 c; 18 a; 19 d; 20 d; 21 a; 22 b; 23 c; 24 b; 25 a

Chapter 4
Dating, Sexual Mores, and Mate Selection

Chapter Outline

American Dating

- American culture is unique in practicing open dating which allows participants to choose their dating partners. Parents often influence dating choices, and they try to influence daughters more than sons.

Why Do We Date?

- The six reasons people date are:
  Recreation
  Status
  Socialization
  Ego
  Mate selection

- As partners continue to date, commitment and intimacy develops toward each other.
- Pressure to engage in sexual relations can adversely affect later relationships especially for young women.

Dating Patterns

- How have dating patterns changed recently:
  (1) Their is greater opportunity for informal opposite sex interaction
  (2) Subsequent dating is less formal
  (3) There no longer seems to be a set of progression of stages

- Traditional, formalized dating has waned, but it is still found in small towns and rural areas.
- Group dating is regaining favor.
- Contrast dating in high school with dating in college: *unwanted sexual contact is reduced*
     High school: *More group dating, group convers., no one on the spot, reduces chances of*
     College: *relaxed, fewer rules, greater diversity of peop., less gossiping about*   *friends assuming a couple is going steady*   *whom is dating*
- There are disadvantages to both going steady or not going steady:
     Going steady: one gains less experience in developing relationships; and one restricts mate choices.
     Not going steady: one may not learn to develop and maintain long and lasting relationships.
- Working out problems during dating is good practice for the give and take of lasting intimate relationships. More experience at dating prevents later problems in marriage.

Dating and Extended Singleness

- Singleness is lasting longer today.
- One in eight adults lived alone in 1990, and the majority were women. Single men tend to be younger on average, 42.5 years old versus 65.8 years old for women.
- First marriages are occurring later in life on average; at age 24.5 years for women and at age 26.5 years for men. The age at first marriage has increased by 4 years for women and 3.3 years for men since 1970.
- Divorces have tripled since 1970.
- Today, forty-two percent of adults are single: 8 % are divorced, 7% are widowed, and 27% have never been married.
- Singleness is considered more acceptable today because:
     The pursuit of personal growth and change has become a more popular goal.
     Our culture has become more tolerant of different lifestyles.
     The women's movement has promoted roles for women other than wife and mother.
     Greater educational opportunities have become available which delay the choice to marry.
     Sexual relationships outside of marriage are increasingly viewed as more acceptable.
- What are the four primary reasons persons remain single?
     wom. want to keep own names
     couples want to keep assets separate
     older people may lose S.S. benefits
     preserve individual status for credit csns, business transactions
- Later marriages have meant:
     Greater risks during pregnancy and birth.
     Greater age differences between parents and children.
     Fewer children in marriages.
     Greater success in marriage.
     Better economic circumstances in beginning the marriage.

- Contrast the advantages and disadvantages of singleness:

  Advantages: _Freedom_   Disadvantages: _loneliness_
  only worry about self   _failure to relate intimately_
  obligations are undertaken voluntarily   _sense of_
  time to do what you want, whenever   _meaninglessness_

- Identify the four types of singles:

  Resolved singles
  Wishful singles
  Ambivalent singles
  Regretful singles

Changing Sexual Mores

- Puberty is the age when youth are first biologically capable of producing children. The average ages for the onset of puberty are _12_ years old for females and _14_ years old for males.
- Therefore, 12 years of singleness occurs on the average for both females and males, and young singles must cope with twelve years of tension as biology allows sexual activity and culture frowns on it.
- Many societal influences encourage sexual activity including the use of makeup and adult fashions, marketing based on sex appeal, and music that promotes themes of sex and drugs.
- The stress of emerging sexuality is compounded by the availability of autos and the ability to be left alone.
- The _female_ (male or female?) usually controls sexual behavior. A double standard that allows sexual activity for males but disapproves of it for females is gradually disappearing.
- From 1965 to 1980, premarital sexual activity increased by 12 % for males and 35% for females.
- Recent studies of sexual activity among teenagers show :

	Men	Women
had sex by age 15	33%	27%
had sex by age 19	86%	80%

- The first sexual partner for women is usually several years older; the first partner for men averages less than 1 year older. The first sexual experience is usually consensual; the earlier the first experience, the more likely it is involuntary.
- While the sexual mores of adults have become less liberal; the mores of youth have become more permissive. However, some youth express the following reasons to abstain from having sex:

  Religious values or one's upbringing and personal code prohibit such behavior.

  Problems may arise from sexual relations such as unwanted children, damaged reputations and psychological problems.

  Premarital sex contributes to the breakdown of the morals of the country.

  Sex is sacred and belongs only in marriage.

  Premarital sex leads to extramarital sex and casual commitment.

  One is more apt to be exposed to sexually transmitted diseases outside of marriage.

Deciding for Yourself

- Identify the four principles couples should examine when contemplating sexual intercourse:

  (1) Personal
  (2) psychological   } 5 PRINCIPLES
  (3) Social
  (4) Religious

Freedom of Choice and Sexual Health

- Is your sexual behavior healthy? Your answer can be explored by asking yourself if your sexual expression enhances your self-esteem, occurs voluntarily, brings enjoyment and gratification, leads to unwanted pregnancies, or passes on sexually transmitted diseases to you or your partner(s)?

Possible Problems Associated with Premarital Sexual Relations

- Identify four problems associated with premarital sexual relations:

  (1) STD's
  (2) Unwanted Pregnancies
  (3) Early commitment
  (4) Isolation, or the quality of sex may be impaired

- The child bearing rate for teenagers was about the same in the 1950's as it is now, but the rate then reflected the lower age of marriage.
- Early commitment based on sex alone is usually an unstable basis for a lasting relationship.
- The quality of sex in early relationships may be impaired because it often occurs under circumstances that arouse fear, conflict or hostility. Thus, later sex life may be crippled.
- The two major reasons for poor premarital sex life are _a negative environment_ and _sexual ignorance of the young couple_
- Relaxation and security are important psychological prerequisites for satisfying sex especially for women.
- Most young women do not enjoy their first sexual encounter which may lead to later problems in attitudes toward sex.

Date Rape and Courtship Violence

- Men and women initiate verbal and physical aggression in about equal numbers.
- Half to three quarters of college women report sexual aggression in a dating relationship.
- Sixty-one percent of rape victims are 17 years old or younger.
- Only 22% of rapes are committed by strangers.
- Misunderstandings about sexual intent are most likely to arise because sexual intentions are not discussed openly and frankly, perceptions of sexual intent differ between partners, token resistance leads to the belief that the protest is token, expectations regarding the stage of the relationship differ between partners, and alcohol and drugs lead to miscommunication.

Finding the One and Only: Mate Selection
- Although love is given as the main reason for marrying, it is complicated and not easily understood.
- Critics argue that compatible social and economic levels, education, age, religion, ethnicity, prior marital experience and race are major factors to consider in mate selection.
- Propinquity: tendency to select mates in the same geographical location and economic class.
- Homogamy: choosing to be with those similar to ourselves based on class, race, religion, etc.
- Endogamy: tendency to marry within our own group.
- Generally, our culture points us to endogamy.

Background Factors
- Generally, the higher the marital quality for parents, the higher the quality of marriage for children.
- Broken homes lead to more complex, stressful and difficult environments and therefore more difficulty in developing satisfactory marital relationships.
- Many studies correlate early marriage with marital instability. Other factors that influence success are age, education, economic class and race.
- Although wives' education seems unrelated to marital stability; educated husbands have more stable marriages than less educated husbands.
- Religious belief /participation and financial success are predictive of marital stability.
- Occupational stress correlates with marriage instability.

Individual Traits
- Personal traits that lead to marital success for both men and women are:
  Good emotional health
  Lack of depression
  Sociability
  +attitudes toward marriage & family
- Impulsiveness negatively influences stability.
- Personality factors generally account for more variance in marital stability than background factors.
- Personality traits and couple interpersonal processes are both important to success in marriage.

Interactional Processes
- Generally, the longer a couple knows one another, the greater the chance of a successful marriage. One to two years appears to be the optimum.
- Miscegenation: prohibition of interracial marriages
- Exogamy: prohibition of marriage to close relatives or to the same sex.
- Two percent of Americans cross racial lines, 20 to 30 percent cross religious lines when marrying.

From First Impression to Engagement

- ___Phys. attractiveness___ tends to create the first appeal, particularly for males.
- Halo effect: first impressions tend to influence succeeding evaluations. Thus, physical attractiveness is a strong asset and is the reason we are so conscious of our body image.
- Women tend to be more dissatisfied with their bodies than men.
- Cognitive compatibility: similarities in thinking, interests, etc. It reinforces our feeling that we are correct and makes us feel good.
- Some marriages do well when partners have similar needs; some do well when partners have complementary needs.

Cohabitation: Unmarried Couple Households

- The number of unmarried couple households increased 400 percent from 1970 to 1993 from 523,000 to 3.5 million. For every 100 married couples, there are 6 unmarried.
- Forty percent of never married women ages 30 to 35 have cohabited.
- Common law marriage: legal change from cohabiting to married after a set number of years.
- Cohabiting couples make up for the lower marriage rate of recent years.
- List four reasons cohabiting is occurring more frequently:
  1. Society's ↑ tolerance toward premarital sexual relations makes cohabitation more acceptable
  2. Higher educ. espec. for wom, ↑ in wom into work force - lessened womens dependence on marriage for econ.
  3. ↑ urbanization leads to ↑ anonymity & ↓ restrictions on individual survival
  4. ↑ levels of divorce may make young people more wary of rushing into marriage

The Nature of Cohabiting Relationships

- List the five reasons couples cohabit:
  1. Short-lived sexual flings
  2. Practical for reasons of expense & safety
  3. Trial marriages
  4. Permenant w/no intent to marry
  5. Fear of marriage & making the same mistake again

Is the Woman Exploited in Cohabitation?

- Only 19 percent of cohabiting men marry their cohabiting partners. More cohabiting women than non-cohabiting women want to marry.
- Cohabiting men are less likely employed; cohabiting women are more likely employed.
- Cohabitants tend to traditionally split chores.
- _____ percent of cohabiting women do not want or enjoy sex with their partners. The rate is higher than for divorced or separated women who had been mistreated.

- Falsehoods:
  - Living together will secure his total commitment.
  - Living together will really help to know one another.
  - Marriage is just a piece of paper.
  - I'm not ready for marriage; I don't want to be alone, and I want to give my love to someone.
- Important questions in considering cohabitation:
  - How did you make the decision to live together?
  - What will you get out of the relationship?
  - What roles do each of you play in the relationship?
  - What were your earlier dating experiences; what did you get from them?
  - What are your partner's primary physical and emotional needs; how will you fulfill them?
  - What are your needs, and how will your partner fulfill them?
  - To what degree do you and your partner honestly share feelings?
  - What are your partner's strengths and weaknesses; how would you change your partner?
  - How do you handle each problem that arises?
  - How will your family and friends react to your living together?

The Relationship Between Cohabitation and Marriage
- There is little relationship between quality of marriage and cohabitation. In fact, some indications show lower quality marriages result. Married cohabits' commitment to the marriage were significantly lower in the first place.
- Higher numbers of cohabitation marriages lead to divorce:
  - Partners learn to withhold commitment in cohabitation.
  - Partners retain a stereotypical romantic ideal of marriage that isn't realized upon marriage.
- Thirty-eight percent of cohabitants, 27 percent of non-cohabitants split up the marriage.
- Divorced persons are more likely to cohabit: 46 percent of women, 56 percent of men. Divorced cohabitants' marriages are more successful than single cohabitants' marriages.
- Cohabiting has little influence on the number of children resulting from the marriage.

Breaking Up
- Forty percent of men, 23 percent of women break up cohabitation within two years. After four years, 75 percent of all couples break up cohabitation.
- Cohabiting break-ups are no less traumatic; yet understanding by others and support systems are not as available to help work through the trauma.

Living Together and the Law
- While some states have laws that forbid cohabitation; the most serious legal consequence is the long term liability e.g. palimony. However, legal protection is limited.

Engagement
- Identify the most important qualities for dates and spouses in rank order:

Dates	Spouse
① Physical Attractiveness	① loving & affectionate
② Congenial Personality	② honest
③ Sense of Humor	③ congenial personality
④ Intelligent	④ Respectful
⑤ Manners/being considerate	⑤ Intelligent
⑥ Sincere, genuine	⑥ Mature/Responsible
⑦ Compatible interests	⑦ Ambitious
⑧ Conversational ability	⑧ Loyal & trustworthy
⑨ fun to be with	⑨ Physical Attractiveness

- Engagement represents a public announcement of your intent to marry. It usually begins the assimilation of partners into each others' families. It begins the treatment of the couple as a pair.

Types of Engagement
- Short, romantic: 2 to 6 months, often couples don't completely develop their relationship before marriage.
- Long, separated: since partners are separated by distance, relationships may not fully develop before marriage.
- Long but inconclusive: putting off the decision, one in four break up temporarily, generally the inability to conclude the marriage signals a lack of commitment.

Function of Engagements
- Engagements should be a time to agree on fundamentals:
    Where will we live?
    How will we live?
    Children?, How many?
    Who works?
    Do our long term goals agree?
    Are our likes and dislikes compatible?
    What are our views on religion?
- The most important agreement may be on how future problems or issues will be resolved by the couple.
- Issues of health and birth control should be fully discussed. Often, discussions with a third party are helpful: e.g. a minister, a marriage counselor, or a friend.

Summary
- American dating has been a unique form of courtship and mate selection.
- Mate selection and sexuality for the young are handled mainly through the American invention of dating.
- Marriage is being postponed, thus increasing the length of time during which a person dates before marriage.
- The onset of puberty signals the beginning of adult sexuality.
- There appears to be increasing acceptance of premarital intercourse in American society.
- Mate selection is an involved process that is not yet fully understood.
- Cohabitation has increased in the past twenty years to such an extent that some theorists now consider it to be a stage in the courtship process.
- Mate selection usually leads to engagement, a formal expression of marital intentions.

Key Terms

1. The five reasons for dating are _Recreation_, _Status_, _Socialization_, _ego_, and _mate selection_.
2. The age at which youth are first capable of bearing children is called _puberty_.
3. As dating continues and leads to marriage, _commitment_ and _intimacy_ are developed in the relationship of young couples.
4. Reasons for remaining single today include _women want to keep their own names_, _couples want to keep assets seperate_ _older peop may lose social security benefits_, and _people want to preserve their own individual status for credit, ins, & business trans_.
5. Individuals who do not want to marry or may not be allowed to marry are called _Resolved singles_.
6. Individuals who are actively searching for a mate are called _wishful singles_.
7. Individuals who would like to marry sometime in the future after they have pursued certain goals or interests are called _ambivalent singles_.
8. Individuals who would like to marry but are stable in their current lifestyle are called _regretful singles_.
9. A set of beliefs that we use to guide our behavior when confronted with issues is referred to as _personal_ _principles_.
10. When personal behavior and attitudes are not congruent, our _psychological_ _principles_ may leave us feeling guilty and stressed.
11. _Social_ _principles_ are those beliefs that society holds as proper behavior.
12. Beliefs passed on to us through religious training are referred to as _Religious principles_.
13. Diseases that are obtained primarily through sexual contact are called _Sexually Transmitted diseases_.
14. Four frequent problems that occur with premarital sexual involvement are _STD's_, _unwanted pregnancies_, _early commitment_, and _isolation or the quality of sex may be impaired_.
15. Adolescent pregnancies are often _unwanted_.
16. Verbal abuse, physical abuse, and sexual abuse that occur during dating are often referred to as _courtship violence_.

17. When individuals marry someone who resides or works in close proximity to them, this is referred to as _propinquity_.

18. Marrying someone of a similar background would be referred to as _endogamy_.

19. Marrying someone within our own group such as race or religion is called _homogamy_.

20. The prohibiting of interracial marriages until 1967 was through _miscengenation_ laws.

21. Requiring people to marry outside their group such as gender is referred to as _exogamy_.

22. When positive first impressions tend to influence future evaluations in a positive way, this is referred to as the _halo_ _effect_.

23. Relationships of individuals who live together for a number of years, usually 7, are legally referred to as _common law marriages_.

24. Cohabiting couples view their relationship in five different ways; they are _short lived sexual fling_, _practical for reasons of expense & safty_, _trial marriages_, _permanent w/no intent to marry_, and _fear of marriage & making the same mistake again_.

25. The type of engagement that typically is very intense and deals mainly with marriage plans is called _short, romantic_.

26. "Absence makes the heart grow fonder" is one philosophy associated with this type of engagement, _long, separated_.

27. An engagement in which marriage is delayed for years due to a variety of reasons is referred to as a _long but inconclusive_.

True-False Questions

1. __F__ Open dating means that parents have no influence on their children's dating choices.
2. __T__ Puberty usually occurs earlier for females than for males.
3. __F__ In the last twenty years, the average age for first marriages has increased more than five years.
4. __T__ The first sexual partner for both men and women is usually older.
5. __T__ Dating and marrying at an early age tends to create unstable marriages.
6. __T__ Recent trends indicate that individuals are dating at earlier ages but marrying at later ages.
7. __T__ In today's society, the norm is to be sexually active.
8. __F__ There are twice as many teenage births today than there were in the 1950's.
9. __F__ Sexual knowledge is especially important in whether women find sexual satisfaction.
10. __F__ Women are more often raped by a stranger than by an acquaintance.
11. __T__ Rape is an act of violence, not a sexual act.
12. __T__ Women with low self-esteem and assertion levels are more often the victims of courtship violence.
13. __F__ Recent studies indicate that women are less committed to their cohabiting partners due to greater gender role equality and emphasis on careers.
14. __F__ Studies indicate that couples who cohabit before marriage are more likely to remain married.
15. __F__ Physical attractiveness is the _most_ important quality given to choose both dates and spouses.
16. __F__ Background factors are more important to marital stability than personality factors.

Multiple-Choice Questions

1. Today, the average time between puberty and marriage for young adults is
    a. three years
    b. five years
    c. ten years
    d. twelve years

2. Marrying later can lead to
    a. greater success in marriage
    b. larger age differences between parents and children
    c. better economic circumstances upon marriage
    d. all of the above

3. Recent studies show that the percentage of nineteen year olds that have been sexually active is
    a. between 25 and 35 percent
    b between 45 and 55 percent
    c. between 60 and 70 percent
    d. between 80 and 90 percent

4. Recent trends in dating indicate
    a. as one progresses through the dating stages, commitment to the relationship decreases.
    b. physical intimacy may occur during any stage while commitment usually progresses in each stage.
    c. physical intimacy occurs in the dating relationship when a firm commitment has been established.
    d. physical intimacy may occur at any time in the dating relationship, while commitment to the relationship comes only when one decides to marry.

5. Which of the following is not a reason for remaining single?
    a. loss of social security benefits
    b. women want to keep their maiden names
    c. preserve standings for credit, insurance, and business transactions
    d. greater number of sexual partners

6. In dating experiences, most individuals face all of the following but one
    a. finding dating partners
    b. coping with bad dates
    c. courtship violence
    d. avoiding exploitation

7. In dating relationships, the person who controls whether sex will occur is
   a. the female
   b. the male
   c. the male and female make the decision jointly
   d. a decision is not made, sex just happens

8. The first sexual experience is often
   a. positive for males and females
   b. positive for males but not for females
   c. positive for females but not males
   d. not positive for either males or females

9. Which of the following is not a characteristic of males who engage in date rape?
   a. value sexuality
   b. have traditional sexual values
   c. view women as property
   d. believe in sexual equality

10. Several studies indicate that one of the following is predictive of marital instability; it is
   a. early age of marriage
   b. wives' education
   c. religious participation
   d. large number of good friends

11. Which of the following statements is true about marital quality?
   a. parents' marital quality does not effect the children's marital quality.
   b. the higher the parents' marital quality, the lower the children's marital quality.
   c. the higher the parents' marital quality, the higher the children's marital quality.
   d. the lower the parents' martial quality, the higher the children's marital quality

12. Generally, the longer a couple knows each other
   a. the lower their chance of a successful marriage because the halo effect wears off
   b. the greater their chance of a successful marriage
   c. the probability for marital success does not change
   d. the lower their chance of marital success due to the influence of background factors

13. Theoretically, the two principles that guide mate selection are
    a. miscegenation and exogamy
    b. endogamy and the halo effect
    c. endogamy and homogamy
    d. endogamy and exogamy

14. All but one are an advantage in the first-impression stage of a relationship:
    a. cognitive compatibility
    b. physical attractiveness
    c. self-disclosure
    d. complementary needs

15. The cohabiting relationship
    a. is no different than marriage in terms of domestic task assignment
    b. exploits men more than women
    c. rarely leads to marriage
    d. none of the above

16. The group most likely to cohabit is
    a. persons who never married
    b. divorced persons
    c. widowed
    d. widowers

17. Which of the following is <u>not</u> one of the falsehoods in cohabiting relationships.
    a. cohabiting will help us get to know each other.
    b. marriage is more than a piece of paper.
    c. cohabiting secures the male's total commitment.
    d. cohabiting will relieve loneliness and give me someone to love.

18. Which of the following is not one of the arguments for cohabitation.
    a. it provides a steady sexual partner and companionship.
    b. it provides a chance for personal growth.
    c. it increases the chance of marital success.
    d. it is a source of financial, social, and emotional security.

19. One reason cohabitation may not lead to a successful marriage is
    a. it teaches the couple to withhold total commitment.
    b. couples tend to take each other for granted over time.
    c. couples lose their romantic ideals about marriage.
    d. none of the above

20. Which statement most accurately represents the dissolution of cohabitation?
    a. it is totally different from the dissolution of a marriage
    b. there is more understanding and support from friends in a cohabiting relationship
    c. cohabiting break-ups are no less traumatic than divorce
    d. dissolution of a cohabiting relationship is relatively easy due to the lack of commitment

21. Which of the following statements reflects parents' and children's attitudes toward mate selection?
    a. the more serious the relationship, the more parents and children try to influence each other.
    b. parents try to influence children but to no avail.
    c. parents try harder to influence their sons' choices.
    d. parents try to influence their children, while children make no effort to influence parents.

22. Dating today has changed from dating of yesteryear in all but one of the following ways.
    a. dating is less formal.
    b. there is no longer a sense of progression from first meeting to marriage.
    c. going steady has declined.
    d. there are more opportunities today for formal interaction.

23. According to the author, the most important thing to remember about dating is
    a. to be most effective, a person must have several partners as well as a wide variety of partners.
    b. courtship must give sufficient experience to make good decisions about intimate relationships.
    c. the number of partners isn't important; most important is the time a couple has known each other.
    d. one dating partner is enough if it is the right one.

24. The optimum time for a couple to get to know each other before marriage is:
    a. six months
    b. one to two years
    c. five years
    d. none of the above

25. Qualities that couple believe are important to mate choice for both dating and marriage include:
  a. wealth
  b. physical attractiveness
  c. coming from a two-parent home
  d. similar strengths and weaknesses

Critical Thinking and Decision Making
1. Discuss why the pressure to have sex is more stressful for young women than for young men.
2. What are the advantages and disadvantages of going steady?
3. Describe your personal, psychological, social and religious principles and how they would affect your choice in engaging in premarital sex. Which do you consider most important? Why?
4. If couples wait to have children at later ages, how will their lives and their relationship with their children be different from parents who have children at younger ages?
5. If engaging in premarital sex is acceptable for you, will you encourage or want your children to engage in it as well? How will you respond if they ask if you engaged in premarital sex?
6. When deciding about premarital sex, which of the four principles (personal, psychological, social, religious) do you consider to be most important? Why?
7. Under what conditions would you consider cohabiting? Why?
8. Describe the most important qualities you would seek in a marriage partner. Why?

Debate the Issues
Should contraceptives be made available to students in the schools? At what age?

Answers

Key Terms: 1   recreation, status, socialization, ego and mate selection
2   puberty
3   commitment and intimacy
4   women want to keep their own names, couples want to keep assets separate, older persons may lose Social Security benefits and persons want to preserve their individual status for credit, insurance and business transactions
5   resolved singles
6   wishful singles
7   ambivalent singles
8   regretful singles
9   personal principles
10   psychological principles
11   social principles
12   religious principles
13   sexually transmitted diseases
14   sexually transmitted diseases, unwanted pregnancies, early commitment and isolation or the quality of sex may be impaired
15   unwanted
16   courtship violence
17   propinquity
18   endogamy
19   homogamy
20   miscegenation
21   exogamy
22   halo effect
23   common law marriages
24   short-lived sexual flings, practical for reasons of expense and safety, trial marriages, permanent with no intent to marry, and fear of marriage and making the same mistake again
25   short, romantic
26   long, separated
27   long but inconclusive

True/False: 1 F; 2 T; 3 F; 4 T; 5 T; 6 T; 7 T; 8 F; 9 F; 10 F; 11 T; 12 T; 13 F; 14 F; 15 F; 16 F

Multiple Choice: 1 d; 2 d; 3 d; 4 b; 5 d; 6 c; 7 a; 8 b; 9 d; 10 a; 11 c; 12 b; 13 c; 14 d; 15 a; 16 b; 17 b; 18 c; 19 a; 20 c; 21 a; 22 d; 23 b; 24 b; 25 b

Chapter 5
Marriage, Intimacy, Expectations, and the Fully Functioning Person

Chapter Outline

- Most adults try to fulfill their psychological, material, and sexual needs within marriage.

<u>Reasons for Marriage</u>
- The key to successful relationships is the couple's learning to _____ and _____ with one another. Marrying to escape home, to simply avoid loneliness, or based on sexual attraction alone usually does not lead to successful relationships.
- More than one person can become a satisfactory and long-lasting partner for an individual.

<u>You and the State: Legal Aspects of Marriage</u>
- In Western societies, the state is interested in supporting a monogamous marriage; assuring that children are born of legally recognized relationships; protecting property and inheritance rights; and preventing unacceptable marriages, such as those between close relatives.
- In the US, marriage laws differ by state. All states recognize marriages contracted in all other states.
- Unlike most contracts, the marriage contract involves three parties: _____ , _____ , and _____. The contract can only be dissolved by state action, not by mutual consent of the man and woman.
- Some states recognize common law marriages if a man and woman have lived together for a prescribed period of time.
- A few cities have set up domestic partnership policies to recognize as valid other hetero- or homosexual couples. Partners may receive medical benefits, sick leave, or bereavement leave based on the relationship.

- Marriage contracts require mutual consent and competency, and usually a prescribed form must be followed. No specific ceremony is required, but the parties must declare in the presence of the person solemnizing the marriage that they take each other as husband and wife, and the marriage must be witnessed, usually by two persons.
- Religious faiths regard marriage as a sacrament, and states vest the clergy with the legal right to perform marriage ceremonies.
- Marriage commits the couple to a new set of obligations and responsibilities prescribed by the state.

The Wedding
- About _____ percent of couples marry in a church.
- Weddings can be expensive. Costs run upwards of $6,000 and can easily reach $10,000 to $15,000.

Writing Your Own Marriage Contract
- Marriage or prenuptial contracts supplement the state marriage contract. They facilitate open and honest communication, help prospective partners clarify their expectations, and guide future behavior.
- Any topics may be covered, but usually marriage contracts cover the following:

    _____
    _____
    _____

    Income and expense handling and control
    Property owned before and acquired after the contract
    Disposition of prior debts
    Living arrangements
    Responsibility for household tasks
    Surname
    Sexual relations
    Relations with family, friends, and others
    Decisions regarding children (number, rearing, etc.)
    Religion
    Inheritance and wills
    Resolving disagreements
    Changing and amending the contract
    Dissolution of the relationship
- It may be worthwhile to discuss the above topics even if a legal written contract is not established. The couple can bring attitudes and expectations into the open and make appropriate compromises and changes before major problems arise.

The Transition from Single to Married Life

- Upon marriage, one becomes interdependent with the other members in the family and loses much of the independence of singleness.
- Couples must work together to live within a family budget and leisure time must be planned with each other.
- Relationships must be developed with both sets of parents.
- Wallerstein and Blakeslee list _____ as one of the essential tasks of a married couple.
- Marriage signals the transition from the _____ of childhood to the _____ of adulthood.

Marriage: A Myriad of Interactions

- Marriage is an arena of intimate and complex interactions. Not only will couples interact as man/woman and husband/wife but also as friends, lovers, provider, provided for, spendthrift, budgeter, father, mother, child, taker, giver, teacher, learner, worker, employer, colleague, tower of strength, and leaning tower. Each partner will take on differing roles in different interactions.

Fulfilling Needs in Marriage

- Society recognizes that fulfilling _____ , _____ , and _____ needs are valid responsibilities of the marriage institution. All states recognize failure to do so as a legitimate reason for divorce.
- Need relationships:
    Psychological needs are closely related to both sexual and material needs.
    The relationship between sexual and psychological needs tends to be more complicated than the relationship between material and psychological needs.
- When other psychological needs are not being met, the _____ relationship is often the first place in which trouble appears. Fewer than 10 percent of successfully married couples believe a good sexual relationship kept their marriages together. However, unhappy couples often list sexual relations as one of their major problems.

Defining Marital Success

- Marital success, defined broadly, includes _____ , _____ , and _____ .
- Marital interaction and partner happiness appear to reciprocally affect each other.
- A definitive list of factors that influence a couple's ability to attain marital success can not be developed; however, the _____ and the _____ relate to lower marital satisfaction.
- Cross-sectional research finds that satisfaction during marriage follows a U-shaped curve, dropping to a low as children reach adolescence in the family and rising during later stages. However, longitudinal research does not support the U-shaped curve. Remarriages follow the same trends.

- Couples probably vary so much that it is difficult to determine how satisfaction is related to the presence of children and to the passage of time.

Strong Relationships and Families

- Stinnett finds that the happiest memories recalled almost always involve _____ .
- Curran states: "lack of time might be the most pervasive enemy the healthy marriage and family have."
- The major revolution in family structure in recent years has been the dual-earner family. Thus, time together has become more scarce. Quality and quantity of time spent together go hand in hand.
- Strong families seem to have the ability to work, play, and vacation together without smothering one another.
- McCubbin finds that almost all strong families reserve one meal a day as a time for family togetherness.
- If the desire to spend time together can be expanded from the time couples are newly in love throughout the marriage, then a key element to maintaining family growth and stability is in place.

Marital Expectations

- _____ _____ play an important role in achieving family success.
- The study of how people experience their world is called _____ .
- Most people react to their perceptions of the world rather than to what the world really is.
- A myth is a belief held uncritically and without examination. Some popular American myths include:
    (False) A husband's marital satisfaction is usually lower if his wife is employed full-time than if she is a full-time homemaker.
    (True) Today most young, single, never-married people will eventually get married.
    (False) In most marriages having a child improves marital satisfaction for both spouses.
    (____) The best single predictor of overall marital satisfaction is the quality of a couple's sex life.
    (True) The divorce rate in America increased between 1960 and 1980.
    (True) A greater percentage of wives are in the work force today than in 1970.
    (False) Marital satisfaction for the wife is usually lower if she is employed than if she is a full-time homemaker.
    (____) If my spouse loves me, he/she should instinctively know what I want and need to be happy.
    (False) In a marriage in which the wife is employed full time, the husband usually assumes an equal share of the housekeeping.
    (False) For most couples, marital satisfaction gradually increases from the first year of marriage through the childbearing years, the teen years, the empty nest period, and retirement.
    (False) No matter how I behave, my spouse should love me simply because he or she is my spouse.
    (____) One of the most frequent marital problems is poor communications.
    (False) Husbands usually make more lifestyle adjustments than wives.
    (____) Couples who have cohabited before marriage usually report greater marital satisfaction than those who did not.
    (False) I can change my spouse by pointing out her or his inadequacies, errors, and so forth.

(True) Couples who marry when one or both partners are under the age of eighteen have more chance of eventually divorcing than those who marry when they are older.

(False) Either my spouse loves me or does not love me; nothing I do will affect the way my spouse feels about me.

(False) The more a spouse discloses positive and negative information to her or his partner, the greater the marital satisfaction of both partners.

(False) I must feel better about my partner before I can change my behavior toward her or him.

(____) Maintaining romantic love is the key to marital happiness over the life span for most couples.

The Honeymoon is Over: Too High Expectations

- "The honeymoon is over" means that partners are reexamining their unrealistic, overly high expectations about marriage and their mate created by "romantic love".
- Partners' ideals and reality seldom coincide exactly and disappointment is almost inevitable.
- Realizing the humanness of our partners allows us to relax and be human as well.
- If expectations are _____ , _____ , or _____ , one can feel betrayed even if one hasn't been. Couples must share their expectations with one another.

Romantic Love or Marriage?

- Physical longing is a tension between desire and fulfillment. When sexual desire is fulfilled, romantic love changes to a feeling of affection that is more durable, though less intense and frenzied, than romantic love.

Differing Expectations

- In a culture in which roles are clearly specified, couples find it easy to define what a good spouse is. When role specification is left to the individual couple, confusion may occur.

80 Percent I Love You : 20 Percent I Dislike You

- The expectation of total need fulfillment within marriage ruins many marital relationships. With time, a spouse will accuse her/his partner of failure and indifference to unmet needs.

Lack of Commitment: Too Low Expectations

- All studies on successful marriages find commitment to the permanence of the relationship is high on the list of reasons couples give for marital success.
- Commitment is often absent in cohabitation. It may be this element that makes cohabitation less than good training for marriage.

The Expectation of Commitment: A Characteristic of Strong and Successful Families
- _____ is the single strongest factor influencing the success of a relationship.

- Commitment is multi-faceted:
    Commitment to a partner to overcome problems and strengthen a relationship.
    Commitment to the family unit to support, love, and affirm each other.
- Facets of commitment:
    long-lasting, provides stability
    overrides all other commitments, even to work
- Individuation: individual family members are encouraged to have independent thoughts, feelings, and judgments.
- Curran found that healthy families exhibit a _____ .
- Commitment has many sides: _____ , _____ , _____ , acceptance, belonging, love, and enduring concern about each other's personal well-being.

The Expectation of Primariness: Extramarital Relations
- _____ percent of all Americans believe in faithfulness in marriage.
- In Kinsey's studies in the late 1940's and early 1950's, 26 percent of women and 34 percent of men were unfaithful.
- With the sexual revolution, sociologists felt the percentages increased considerably. Yet recent studies in 1994 by Michael show that 20 percent of women and 15 to 35 percent of men had other sexual partners while married. Studies in 1995 by Wallerstein and Blakeslee report 16 percent of women and 20 percent of men had brief affairs while married.
- Working wives have a _____ incidence of extramarital relations than housewives.
- Greater acceptance of extramarital affairs correlates with being: _____ , _____ , _____ , _____ , egalitarian toward gender roles, politically liberal, unmarried, and premaritally sexually permissive.
- Generally speaking, _____ tend to regard extramarital affairs more lightly than _____ because women tend to be more emotionally involved in sexual relationships. Grosskopf report 72 percent of women give _____ as the major reason for an affair.
- Extramarital affairs damage trust, and trust is the cornerstone of a lasting and enduring relationship.

The Self-Fulfilling Prophecy
- Persons tend to live up to expectations. However, impossible expectations lead to feelings of _____ , _____ , and _____ .

The Self-Actualized Person in the Fully Functioning Family
- Healthy, intimate marriages require psychologically healthy partners.

<u>Characteristics of Mental Health</u>
- A mentally healthy person:
  - Feels comfortable with her/himself
  - Feels good about other people
  - Feels competent to meet the demands of life

<u>Self-Actualization</u>
- Self-actualized people have reached the highest levels of growth, are realizing their full potential, have achieved the highest mental health, and can create successful intimate relationships:
- The characteristics of self-actualized persons are:

  _____

  _____

  _____

  Focus on problem-centeredness
  Need privacy
  Exhibit a high degree of autonomy
  Have a continued freshness of appreciation

<u>Living in the Now</u>
- Retention and projection of time can help us cope with the present, but it can also hamper present behavior.

<u>The Goals of Intimacy</u>
- The goals of intimacy are identical to some of the functions of the family. They involve:

  _____

  _____

  _____

<u>Summary</u>
- Marriage is a three-way relationship involving the man, the woman, and the state.
- The marriage ceremony commits a couple to a new status, with certain privileges, obligations, and restrictions.
- Marriage is constant interaction between family members and fulfillment of many roles within the family relationship.
- Expectations that are too high or too low can lead to relationship problems.
- Self-actualizing people feel comfortable about themselves and others and are able to meet most demands of life in a realistic fashion.
- The basic goals of intimacy in a marriage are providing emotional gratification to each partner, helping each deal with crises, and helping each grow in a fulfilling manner.

Key Terms

1. A written agreement by a marrying couple that delineates responsibilities and obligations of each person is called a _____.
2. A responsibility of marriage is to fulfill _____, _____, and _____ needs of each individual.
3. In broad terms, marital success includes _____, _____, and _____.
4. The study of how people experience their world is called _____.
5. Having independent thoughts, feelings, and judgments is referred to as _____.
6. Mentally healthy people generally possess three characteristics: _____, _____, and _____.

True-False Questions

1. _____ A fully functioning family helps its members grow, mature, and become self-actualized individuals.
2. _____ The better the marriage, the more it protects its members from mental health problems such as alienation, loneliness, and depression.
3. _____ The key to a successful relationship is communication and learning to compromise.
4. _____ Terms set forth in prenuptial contracts can override a state marriage contract.
5. _____ One advantage of having a prenuptial contract is the increased predictability and security of helping couples identify and resolve potential conflicts in advance.
6. _____ Failure to meet spouses sexual, material, and psychological needs are recognized as legitimate reasons for divorce.
7. _____ When psychological needs are not being met, the sexual relationship is often the first area that is affected negatively.
8. _____ Research indicates that marital satisfaction decreases as children enter the home and increases when children leave the home.
9. _____ One major characteristic of a strong, resilient family is the desire to spend time together.
10. _____ Many people expect their spouses to meet all of their needs, however, it is impossible for one person to meet all the needs of another.
11. _____ Truly loving another person allows them to see all of their partners faults.
12. _____ Housewives have a higher incidence of extramarital affairs.
13. _____ The single strongest factor influencing the success of a relationship is commitment to the relationship and the partner.

Multiple-Choice Questions
1. Which is not one of the primary functions of the American family?
    a. providing emotional gratification
    b. helping members deal with emotional crisis
    c. providing status and roles
    d. helping members become self-actualized

2. All marriage contracts must
    a. be entered into by mutual consent
    b. follow a prescribed form
    c. be completed by individuals competent and eligible to enter into the contract
    d. all of the above

3. What percentage of people marry in a church?
    a. 75%
    b. 50%
    c. 90%
    d. 85%

4. Which is not one of the items necessary for a successful marriage?
    a. pulling together rather than in opposite directions
    b. to always compromise when a disagreement arises
    c. to consider the likes and dislikes of one's partner
    d. to realize that the pair as a whole is greater than the two individuals

5. Research indicates that two factors closely relate to marital satisfaction and success?
    a. number of children and degree of conflict
    b. age at marriage and presence of children
    c. adjustment to roles and liking one's spouse
    d. agreeing on important issues and adjustment to the relationship

6. According to Curran, the most pervasive enemy of a healthy marriage and family is
    a. romantic love
    b. women in the labor force
    c. stereotypic roles of men and women
    d. lack of time together

7. Which of the following is true?
    a. having a child improves marital satisfaction for both spouses
    b. husband's marital satisfaction is usually lower if his wife is employed full time
    c. the younger a couple is at marriage, the more likely they are to divorce
    d. the best single predictor of overall marital satisfaction is the quality of a couple's sex life

8. One of the greatest disappointments newly married couples face is
    a. the fading of romantic love
    b. decreasing sexual interest
    c. decreased contact with parents
    d. none of the above

9. Commitment in a strong family is multifaceted. Which is not one of those discussed by the author?
    a. commitment to partner and family as a whole
    b. commitment to parental values
    c. commitment to family overrides all other commitments
    d. commitment is long-lasting

10. Which statement best summarizes the research on the occurrence of extramarital affairs?
    a. about half of all Americans believe in fidelity and practice it
    b. infidelity has increase over the years and recent research indicates that 50% of all marriages
       experience an extramarital affair
    c. most Americans believe in fidelity but research indicates that over 50% of marriages experience
       infidelity
    d. recent research indicates that approximately 80% of men and women believe in and practice fidelity

11. When a person holds expectations about another person that tends to influence that person in the
    directions of the expectations, this is called
    a. disappointment
    b. degree of acceptance
    c. the self-fulfilling prophecy
    d. self-actualization

12. In order to have a healthy, intimate marriage, one needs to
    a. admit error and failure
    b. accept criticism
    c. respect and like oneself
    d. all of the above

13. The National Association for Mental Health describes mentally healthy people as having all of the following characteristics but one, it is
    a. feeling comfortable about themselves
    b. underestimating their shortcomings
    c. feeling good about other people
    d. being able to meet the demands of life

14. Feeling competent to meet the demands of life means that people do all of the following but one.
    a. accept responsibilities
    b. welcome new experiences
    c. live for the day
    d. set realistic goals

15. Self-actualized people demonstrate all of the following characteristics but one
    a. have a high need for privacy
    b. have adequate perceptions of reality
    c. have a high degree of spontaneity
    d. are problem centered

16. Marriage contracts involve three parties; which is not one of those parties?
    a. the federal government
    b. the man
    c. the woman
    d. the state

17. A domestic partnership ordinance is
    a. a document agreed to by those who live in a commune
    b. another name for marriage
    c. a legal recognition of cohabitation
    d. a law against mate swapping

18. One advantage of a prenuptial agreement is
    a. it is always legally binding
    b. it facilitates open and honest communication
    c. it tells each partner what he/she can and cannot do
    d. there are not advantages, if two people need a contract, they shouldn't get married

19. Society recognizes that fulfilling certain needs is a responsibility of marriage. Which is not one of those needs?
    a. sexual needs
    b. psychological needs
    c. material needs
    d. social needs

20. Marital disruption tends to be the highest among
    a. the wealthy
    b. middle class
    c. the materially least well-off
    d. none of the above

21. When couples adjust to the relationship, agree on important issues, are comfortable in their roles, and work together to solve problems, this is called
    a. marital permanence
    b. marital success
    c. marital reciprocity
    d. marital adjustment

22. Which statement best describes the relationship between quality and quantity of couple interaction?
    a. as quantity increases, quality decreases
    b. as quality increases, quantity decreases
    c. as quantity increases, quality increases
    d. there is no relationship between the two

23. The phrase "the honeymoon is over" refers to which of the following statements?
    a. partners are reexamining their unrealistic and overly high expectations about marriage and their mate
    b. romantic love has been destroyed
    c. divorce is inevitable
    d. couples intimacy decreases due to work and home demands

24. Which is not one of the factors related to greater acceptance of extramarital affairs?
    a. being politically liberal
    b. being highly educated
    c. being unmarried
    d. being female

25. In Grosskopf's study, the reason most women gave for having an extramarital affair was
   a. their husbands were having affairs
   b. they were emotionally dissatisfied with their husbands
   c. greater desire for sexual companionship
   d. simple curiosity

Critical Thinking and Decision Making
1. Would you create a prenuptial contract if you were about to marry? Why?
2. If you were to create a prenuptial contract, what would you include?
3. Think about strong marital relationships you have observed; what characteristics did they possess that made them strong?
4. What expectations do you hold for your marriage? Why?
5. Identify four myths that people hold about marriage.
6. Do you consider yourself to be a self-actualized person? Why?

Examining International Families
1. Why do Japanese couples put forth one image in public and a different one in the home?
2. Throughout America's history, people have not always married for love and intimacy. Is Japan's system better? Will they eventually change as did America?

Debate the Issues
1. Do you think marriages and families are dying institutions? Why or why not? How would you respond to someone who holds the opposite beliefs?
2. Do you and most of your peers want to marry and have a family?
3. Are the variety of family forms positive for individuals?

Answers

Key Terms: 1   prenuptial contract
2   sexual, material, psychological
3   adjustment, happiness, permanence
4   phenomenology
5   individuation
6   feeling comfortable about oneself, feeling good about other people, able to meet the demands of life

True/False: 1 T; 2 T; 3 T; 4 F; 5 T; 6 T; 7 T; 8 T; 9 T; 10 T; 11 F; 12 F; 13 T

Multiple Choice: 1 c; 2 d; 3 a; 4 b; 5 b; 6 d; 7 c; 8 a; 9 b; 10 d; 11 c; 12 d; 13 b; 14 c; 15 a; 16 a; 17 c; 18 b; 19 d; 20 c; 21 b; 22 c; 23 a; 24 d; 25 b

Chapter 6
Communication in Intimate Relationships

Chapter Outline

- The more intimate the relationship, the more important high-quality communication becomes. Good communication skills are always evident in strong families.

<u>Good Communication: A Basic Strength of Successful Families</u>
- Successful communication is the cornerstone of any relationship.
- Conflict management is essential to all intimate relationships.
- General social values about masculinity and femininity affect marital communication. American men are taught to disclose less about their feelings; women are taught expressiveness, sensitivity, and tenderness.
- Part of good communication is a couple's ability to relate to one another in a manner relatively free from cultural differences.
- McGinnis found that the average couple spent only _seventeen min_ a week in conversation.
- When both partners work, two important factors, _time spent together_ and _conversation_, tend to be weakened.
- Factors that relate to communication skills: _trusting & confiding in one another, trying new ways to deal w/probs_ , _working together to solve probs_, expressing caring and affection for each other daily, at least one family member talking to his or her parents daily, sharing feelings and concerns with close friends, and checking in and out with each other.
- Poor communication leads family members to a feeling of frustration, of not feeling understood, and of not getting their message across. This frustration usually leads to the need to go out, to be constantly on the phone, to have the television set on all the time, or to have headphones in place during family time.
- Poor communication is often evidenced in sharp words, quarrels, and misunderstandings.

What Causes Communication Failure?

- Interpersonal communication: communication with others.
- Intrapersonal communication: communication with ourselves.
- Failure to communicate well with others sometimes begins with a breakdown of intrapersonal communication. When individuals' self-images become unrealistic, they tend to filter all communications to fit the faulty self-picture. Blind spots and overly strong defenses about ourselves interfere with good communication with others.
- Silence is a form of communication that sends a surplus of negative and aversive messages that hasten the disintegration of the relationship.

Aversive Communication

- People first seek to avoid pain and then seek pleasure.
- Responding to a partner who is giving us pain with aversive communication, in turn, threatens the partner and leads to a vicious circle to greater and greater aversive communication.
- Negative thoughts must be communicated, but they must be communicated in positive ways.
  As one becomes aware of negative responses in your interactions with your partner, one should substitute more positive responses to show that you care about your partner and your relationship.

Communication Can Be Used For Good And Bad Purposes

- Good purposes: express honest feelings , convey facts & observations , share helpful info , and enhance another person, ourselves or relationship .
- Bad purposes: manipulate feelings , convey falsehoods , hide info , and degrade another person, ourself relationship .

The Foundation Blocks of Successful Communication

- Three general conditions must be met to achieve the kind of communication that builds strong, positive relationships: commitment , growth orientation , and noncoercive atmosphere .
- Commitment means making a pledge or binding yourself to your partner and includes the idea of working to build and maintain the relationship.
- An individual oriented to growth incorporates the inevitability of change into his or her lifestyle.
- In a noncoercive atmosphere, partners feel free to be themselves, to be open, and to be honest.
- A marriage can be described as:
    laissez-faire if both partners have total freedom of choice and action,
    democratic if responsibility is shared and authority is delegated by equitable agreement, or
    autocratic if both have responsibilities but authority is assigned to a single leader.
- Most Americans want a democratic marriage, but it is the most difficult to maintain.
  In an autocratic marriage, a coercive relationship is usually the result (feeling the loss of freedom).

Developing a Smooth Flow of Communication
- Steps in communication:
  Encode the message and send it to the receiver via some verbal, nonverbal, or written communication channel.
  The receiver decodes the message and must feed back what has been decoded to the sender to ensure that it has been correctly received.
  The sender either verifies the message or through correction, negotiation, and problem-solving, resends the message.

Communication Skills
- The best time to build communication skills is when _disruptive forces are minimal_.
- Clarifying responsibility or problem ownership is an important first step in problem-solving communication. A person must know and openly admit that he or she is personally disturbed by a problem to own or share ownership of it. One must be tangibly affected by a problem to own it.
- American society often encourages individuals to deny ownership by supplying scapegoats or encouraging individuals to claim victimization.
- _Self assertion_ is the process of recognizing and expressing one's feelings, opinions, and attitudes while remaining aware of the feelings and needs of others.
- If persons are nonassertive, successful communication is almost impossible.
- You, I, and We statements:
  _I_ statements are less apt to provoke resistance, are less threatening, and are more effective.
  _WE_ statements place the problem in the group or relationship rather than on one of the individuals.
  You statements are probably least effective in problem-solving situation.
- Successful communication in large part depends on knowing oneself. The Johari window diagrams what we and others know or don't know about ourselves. As relationships grow, partners usually learn more about themselves and each other.

Empathic Listening
- _Empathy_ means not only understanding what the speaker is saying but also being able to respond to and feel the speaker's nonverbal communications and emotions.
- Being a good listener is an art, is much appreciated by most people, and is one of the most important ingredients of intimate relationships.
- Empathic listening is nonjudgemental and accepting.
- Selective _Attention_ filters out what we do not want to hear.
- Selective _retention_ remembers only what one want to remember.
- Nonverbal communication is often referred to as _body language_ and usually represents a more accurate picture of how a person is feeling emotionally than verbal communication. People in good marriages read it as well as words.
- The more intimate a relationship, the closer persons can physically be and feel comfortable.

- Research shows: nonverbal communication is subject to many interpretations; when verbal and nonverbal communication conflicts, the _nonverbal_ meaning tends to be believed; and unhappy partners tend to read nonverbal communication more negatively than happy partners.
- Empathic listeners provide feedback by periodically checking their perceptions with the speaker by paraphrasing the speaker's words.
- Pearson suggests six behaviors to facilitate feedback: _Provide clear verbal feedback_; rely on descriptive statements; _Provide reflective statements_; demonstrate bodily responsiveness; use a sincere, warm voice; and _Establish eye contact_.
- The desire to give advice is a major deterrent to empathic listening. Offering alternatives is a better way of providing feedback.
- Negotiation is required when a problem is jointly owned. It requires partners to alternate between self-assertion and empathic listening.
- The seven stages of scientific problem-solving: _Recognize & define problem_; set up conditions supportive to problem solving; _Brain storm for possible alternatives / Establish hypothesis_; select the best solution; implement the solution; evaluate the solution; and modify the solution if necessary.

Men and Women: Do They Speak the Same Language?
- In general, men grow up in a competitive world in which independence is the key.
- In general, women grow up in a world of connection in which intimacy is the key.
- Women believe it is natural to consult their partners often while men automatically make more decisions without consultation.

Communication and Family Conflict
- Conflicts are equally present in happy and unhappy marriages. The difference is that partners in happy marriages learn how to handle conflicts and even use them to improve their relationship.
- _Realistic_ conflict results from frustration over specific needs. _Nonrealistic_ conflict results from the need to release tension by at least one of the partners.
- _Hidden_ conflict relies on one of the following communication strategies: Denial, disqualification, displacement, disengagement, or pseudomutuality.
- The chances of dealing with conflict are _greater_ (greater or less) if it is overt rather than covert.
- Verbal abuse can cause real psychological damage if it is extended over a long period of time. Physical violence seldom solves a conflict.
- Areas of conflict fall in six clusters: _power_, social issues, _personal flaws_, distrust, intimacy, and personal distance.
- Conflicts over partners' jobs tend to diminish over time. Conflicts over household tasks and partners' friends, particularly the husbands', tend to increase over time.

Summary
- Good communication is one of the major characteristics of strong, successful families.
- Society can facilitate or hinder good communication.
- Failure in communication for most people means that communication has become so aversive that it causes discomfort.
- Three basic conditions must be met for good communication to be assured: commitment, growth orientation, and noncoercive atmosphere.
- Five skills are involved in successful problem-solving communication; identifying ownership, self-assertion, empathic listening, negotiation, and willingness to use problem-solving methods.
- Using problem-solving skills and avoiding both physical and verbal abuse will enhance any relationship and keep it alive and growing.

Key Terms

1. _Commitment_ means making a pledge to your partner to build and maintain the relationship.
2. Partners who believe that their relationship will always be dynamic and changing rather than static are said to have a _growth orientation_ attitude.
3. When partners feel free to be themselves and to be open and honest, they have created a _noncoersive_ atmosphere.
4. A marriage in which both partners have total freedom of choice and action is called _laissez-faire_.
5. When responsibility is shared and authority is delegated by equitable agreement, the relationship is _democratic_.
6. When both partners have responsibilities but authority is assigned to one person, the relationship is _autocratic_.
7. The process of sending a communication is _encoding_, _comm. channel_, _decoding_, and _feedback_.
8. A sender verifies a message through _correction_, _negotiation_, and _prob. solving_.
9. The process of recognizing and expressing one's feelings, opinions, and attitudes while remaining aware of the feelings and needs of others is called _self assertion_.
10. "You never listen to me" is an example of a _you statement_.
11. "We don't spend time together like we once did" is an example of a _we statement_.
12. "I need more affection" is an example of an _I statement_.
13. We-statements are used when one wants to enhance the _togetherness_ aspect of the relationship.
14. The _Johari Window_ is a way of looking at the known and unknown dimensions of the self.

15. People use ___selective atten___ when they want to filter out what they do not want to hear.
16. Remembering only what one wants to remember about a conversation is called
    ___selective retention___.
17. Nonverbal communication is also called ___body lang___.
18. In the world of status, ___independence___ is the key.
19. For women, ___intimacy___ is the key in the world of connection.
20. ___Denial___ is refusing to admit there is a problem.
21. Expressing anger and then discounting it is called ___disqualification___.
22. Avoiding conflict by avoiding one another is called ___disengagement___.
23. Giving the appearance of being perfectly happy and delighted with one's partner is called
    ___Pseudomutuality___.
24. Placing emotional reactions somewhere other than the real source is called ___displacement___.
25. The sending and receiving of verbal or nonverbal messages is called
    ___communication___.

True-False Questions

1. ___F___ If two people truly love each other and have good communication skills, conflict will not arise nor will anger.
2. ___T___ A major problem almost always cited by couples who are experiencing marital difficulties is failure to communicate.
3. ___T___ Each person brings communication and conflict resolution skills to a relationship - good or bad.
4. ___T___ Silence can communicate just as much as verbal communication can.
5. ___T___ Communication is a double-edged sword. It can improve a relationship or it can destroy it.
6. ___T___ Most marriages end up being a mixture of laissez-faire, democratic, and autocratic.
7. ___F___ Sharing responsibilities, giving up control voluntarily, and feeling free in a relationship hinders communication because over time people feel that they have given up too much independence.
8. ___T___ The first step toward conflict resolution is problem ownership.
9. ___F___ What one says when communicating is more important than how one conveys his/her views.
10. ___F___ We-statements place the responsibility for the problem on both people but assigns more responsibility to one than the other.
11. ___F___ When verbal and nonverbal communication are in disagreement, the more accurate perception can be derived through verbal communication.
12. ___T___ Good listeners periodically check their perceptions with paraphrasing.
13. ___T___ The desire to give advice is one of the major deterrents to empathic listening and clear feedback.

Multiple-Choice Questions

1. Without the following there would be no relationship.
   - a. sex
   - b. communication
   - c. love
   - d. sharing

2. Curran identified which two traits as primary to healthy families?
   - a. conflict and communication
   - b. conflict and problem solving skills
   - c. communication and listening
   - d. intimacy and communication

3. When both partners work outside the home, what two important factors tend to be weakened?
   - a. time spent together and conversation
   - b. problem solving skills and communication
   - c. intimacy and shared leisure activities
   - d. time spent with children and conflict

4. The key to a successful relationship is
   - a. sharing responsibilities
   - b. sharing leisure activities
   - c. positive communication
   - d. intimacy

5. Which of the following is not a general condition for achieving strong, positive relationships?
   - a. commitment
   - b. growth orientation
   - c. noncoercive atmosphere
   - d. pseudomutuality

6. The principle of least interest means
   - a. the one least interested in the relationship will care the most
   - b. the one who cares the least has the most power
   - c. the person least interested in the relationship will become resentful of the other person's attitude
   - d. none of the above

7. Which is not one of the types of marital responsibility and authority?
    a. autocratic
    b. authoritarian
    c. laissez-faire
    d. democratic

8. Putting information in a sendable form and identifying problem ownership is called
    a. encoding
    b. channeling
    c. decoding
    d. feedback

9. Which of the following is least effective in problem-solving situations?
    a. I-statements
    b. we-statements
    c. they-statements
    d. you-statements

10. Which of the following is not characteristic of I-statements?
    a. they are less threatening
    b. they locate feelings or concerns inside the person
    c. they tend to place blame
    d. they may contain "feeling," "when," and "because" parts

11. Which statement is false about we-statements?
    a. they increase the imbalance of power
    b. they tend to reduce emotional distance
    c. they emphasize togetherness
    d. problem solving is directed at both partners

12. Which of the following is not one of the components of the Johari Window?
    a. unknown to self
    b. secrets told to one person
    c. known to self and others
    d. my blind spots

13. "Hearing only what one wants to hear" is an example of
    a. selective retention
    b. displacement
    c. disqualification
    d. selective attention

14. In reviewing the literature on nonverbal communication, L'Abate and Bagarozzi found all of the following but one:
    a. unhappy partners tend to read nonverbal communications negatively more often than happy couples
    b. nonverbal communication is subject to many interpretations
    c. nonverbal messages give little insight into problems
    d. when verbal and nonverbal messages conflict, the nonverbal tends to be believed

15. Which of the following statements is false about women's communication skills?
    a. stereotypic women seek marriage in order to find intimacy and commitment
    b. women expect decisions to be discussed and made by consensus
    c. women feel it is natural to consult their partners at every turn
    d. women always talk more than men

16. Which of the following is false about men's communication skills?
    a. men try to avoid marriage in order to preserve their independence
    b. men tend to back away from making decisions that involve the marriage
    c. men make more decisions without consultation
    d. men feel oppressed by lengthy discussions

17. Men and women can communicate better if
    a. men would use more eye contact
    b. women would discuss issues concerning the present and not the past
    c. women would not nag men into opening up
    d. all of the above

18. Phyllis is very upset with Debra, but yells at her daughter, Tisha; this is an example of
    a. displacement
    b. disengagement
    c. pseudomutuality
    d. disqualification

19. Successful conflict management can be described as
    a. sequential communication exchange
    b. partners respecting differences of opinions
    c. controlling television watching
    d. all of the above

20. In Lawrence Kurdek's study of conflict in gay, lesbians, and heterosexual relationships, he found
    a. heterosexual couples argue more about intimacy
    b. heterosexual couples argue more about social issues
    c. gay and lesbian couples argue more about social issues
    d. gay and lesbian couples argue more about personal flaws

21. McCubbin found many factors that are related to communication skills, which is not one of those skills?
    a. trust
    b. sharing feelings and concerns with close friends
    c. attending communication seminars
    d. trying new ways to deal with problems

22. Which of the following is a positive response in communication?
    a. providing self-direction and choice
    b. analyzing and diagnosing
    c. probing, questioning, and interrogating
    d. giving solutions or suggestions

23. A vital component of the communication process is
    a. encoding
    b. decoding
    c. feedback
    d. channeling

24. In the communication process, one skill that is very important yet often very difficult to achieve, is
    a. self-disclosure
    b. being a good listener
    c. decision making
    d. selective attention

25. The primary complaint of many wives who seek marital counseling is
    a. lack of intimacy
    b. being primarily responsible for children and the home
    c. husbands who nag
    d. withdrawn, noncommunicative husbands

Critical Thinking and Decision Making

1. On a scale of 1 to 10 how would you rate your conflict resolution abilities. Why?
2. Explain how communication can hinder or promote a relationship.
3. How honest are you when dealing with other people in relationships? Do you not say anything to avoid a conflict or so you won't hurt anyone's feelings? How often do you do this?
4. Think about the relationships you have had. Have they been primarily autocratic, democratic, or laissez-faire? Why?
5. Referring to Table 6-1, do you give more negative or positive responses during communication?

Answers

Key Terms:
1	commitment
2	growth orientation
3	noncoercive
4	laissez-faire
5	democratic
6	autocratic
7	encoding, communication channel, decoding, feedback
8	correction, negotiation, problem-solving
9	self-assertion
10	you-statement
11	we-statement
12	I-statement
13	togetherness
14	Johari Window
15	selective attention
16	selective retention
17	body language
18	independence
19	intimacy
20	denial
21	disqualification
22	disengagement
23	pseudomutuality
24	displacement
25	communication

True/False: 1 F; 2 T; 3 T; 4 T; 5 T; 6 T; 7 F; 8 T; 9 F; 10 F; 11 F; 12 T; 13 T

Multiple Choice: 1 b; 2 c; 3 a; 4 c; 5 d; 6 b; 7 b; 8 a; 9 d; 10 c; 11 a; 12 b; 13 d; 14 c; 15 d; 16 b; 17 d; 18 a; 19 d; 20 b; 21 c; 22 a; 23 c; 24 b; 25 d

Chapter 7
Role Equity: The Converging of the Sexes

Chapter Outline

- Gender role: culturally assigned behaviors based on a person's gender.

Role Equity

- When men and women are freer to choose gender roles for themselves their chances for success and fulfillment increase. In intimate relationships, satisfaction is greater if partners can share the decisions and responsibilities they feel right for them than if they are forced into stereotyped behaviors that may not fit.
- Role equity means that roles are based on individual _strengths_ and _weaknesses_ rather than on preordained stereotypical differences based on the sexes.
- _Androgyny_ means the blending of traits associated with the sexes. Equity focuses on gender role transcendence.

Male = Masculine and Female = Feminine: Not Necessarily So

- Gender identity is how one views one's self; am I masculine or feminine?
- One's sex is biologically determined; am I male or female?
- Gender not only includes biological sex but all of the attitudes and behaviors that are expected of that sex by a given society.

Norms and Roles

- Norms are accepted and expected patterns of _behaviors_ and _beliefs_ established either formally or informally by a group.
- In the United States, sanctions against cross-gender behavior are greater for boys than for girls.

- Roles involve activities demanded by the norms. Because there are many norms in a society, a person plays many roles.
- Problems occur when roles and norms are not accepted or when they are unclear.
- In American society, almost all norms and roles are being questioned.

How Sex and Gender Identity Develops

- Gender identity is determined by three factors:
  - <u>Genetics</u> determine sex at conception.
  - <u>hormones</u> determined by genetics produce physical differences.
  - <u>Society</u> defines, prescribes, and reinforces gender roles.

Biological Contributions

- Every normal person has two sex chromosomes; women have two X chromosomes, men have an X and a Y chromosome. Either the father's X or Y chromosome combines with the mother's X chromosome to determine the sex of the child.
- The presence of the male hormone <u>testosterone</u> causes the embryo to develop male organs. In the absence of the hormone, female organs are developed.
- During puberty, increases in <u>hormonal activity</u> and ~~female phase~~ (estrogen) occur in females, and increases in testosterone occur in males.
- Both sexes produce male and female hormones; the direction of development is determined by the balance of the hormones.
- <u>hermaphrodites</u>: rare cases when the hormones fail to set a sexual direction in an individual.
- <u>Transexual</u> : a person who feels psychologically that he or she is of the opposite gender.
- <u>Transvestite</u> : a person who gains sexual pleasure from dressing like the opposite sex.

Environmental Contributions

- Cultures exhibit different attitudes and expect different behaviors in the sexes.
- Children learn sex-appropriate behaviors.
- <u>Sexual identity confusion</u> : a failure to learn the role that traditionally accompanies one's biological sex.

The Theory of Gender Role Development

- Gender roles are determined by the interaction of biological and environmental factors.
- Ullian theorized that sex-appropriate behavior is developed in three stages:
  - Stage 1: <u>Biological</u> Orientation (from birth to ten years) in which biological influence is most clearly seen.
  - Stage 2: <u>Societal</u> Orientation (from ten to fourteen years) in which behavior is more socially influenced.
  - Stage 3: <u>Psychological</u> Orientation: (from fourteen to eighteen years) in which behavior is formed from a personal psychological orientation.

- Studies show that the differences in behavior between persons of the same sex on a given characteristic are greater than the average differences between the sexes.

Traditional Gender Roles

- Traditional roles historically reflect the woman's childbearing function and the man's greater physical strength and his need to support and defend his family.
- The traditional feminine role is essentially the complement of the masculine role.
- Double standard: traditional roles allow men more sexual freedom while limiting severely women's sexuality.
- The reason that the traditional role for women has been found in almost all cultures and throughout history is that women _bear the children_ .
- Traditional _masculine_ character traits are those labeled "instrumental" while _feminine_ traits are those labeled "expressive".

The Feminine Liberation Movement

- The women's movement has focused our attention on gender inequalities and has energized efforts to reduce these inequalities. To the extent that it has succeeded, it has also meant men's liberation.
- The failure of the Equal Rights Amendment, the strength of the prolife attack on abortion, and the antifeminist movement demonstrate the conflicts that are stirred up when traditional gender roles are challenged.

Women and the Law

- In the past, laws have considered females to be weaker and less responsible than men and therefore in need of protection.
- Since the 1970s, many laws have been enacted guaranteeing both women and men more protection against unfair discrimination and unequal treatment.
- Inequities may result as laws are changed to make the sexes more equal. For example, rehabilitative alimony and the Displaced Homemaker's Relief Acts respond to the need for women who have little work experience for greater financial help when divorced.
- Punishment for rape has become more stringent, and some states have eliminated the humiliating defense tactic of cross-examining the victim.
- Women have increasingly won sexual harassment cases.
- Naomi Wolf cites the following as victories women have won as a result of the Thomas-Hill case:
    - The Family Leave Act passed.
    - The Federal budget has been doubled for research on women's health and breast cancer in particular.
    - Antistalking bills were passed.
    - Ruth Bader Ginsburg became the second woman appointed to the US Supreme Court.

Gender Role Stereotypes
- Traditional marriages in which the husband is the primary breadwinner and the wife has primary responsibility for the home and family work well for many couples. However, in such marriages, some men may find this a heavy burden, and some women may come to feel isolated and restricted.
- In a relationship based on equity, each mate must be committed to the idea of seeking equity and to communicating openly any feelings of inequity.

The Movement Toward Gender Equality

from more econ. dependent / men ↓ econ. supp.
* Women are freer sexually / fathers less supportive
* ↑ women working in mngmnt

- Gains for women:

  * more job opportunities / pay differentials still remain.
  * more women in the labor force / low-level jobs.
  * single parent fam headed by women / lgst group below poverty line.

  Maternity leaves, parental leaves, and flexible work schedules are now available.
  Good child care facilities are increasingly recognized as important to families.
  Women's school sports are gaining equality with men's sports.

- Some feminists still cite women's disadvantages:

  _____ .

  _____ .

  Single parent families headed by women have increased greatly in number and make up the largest group below the poverty line.
  The number of children born out of wedlock and not supported by their fathers is larger than ever.
  A " glass ceiling " bars women from the highest levels of management.
  As women have increased their economic support for the family, men have reduced theirs.

- Many women now avoid being labeled a feminists although they supported many of the earlier feminists goals such as better pay, better childcare, and better jobs. Authors cite various reasons for this including the continuing use of vitriolic terms to describe a gender war, the support of lesbians, the support of abortion, and the belittling of motherhood.

The Women's Movement: Some Losses
- Losses to women revolve around sexuality , child bearing , and child rearing .
- Sexual freedom has liberated men, not women. Women complain about finding men who care, who will make commitments, who will respect them, and who will share responsibility for birth control, pregnancy, and their children.
- Statutory rape is seldom prosecuted.
- Child support from divorced fathers has become increasingly difficult to collect.
- Responsibility for children has shifted more and more to women and away from men.

Summary
- Equity between the sexes, not sameness, is the goal to seek.
- Two important stumbling blocks to people's liberation caused by stereotypical gender roles are the economic deprivation of women and laws that discriminate between the sexes.
- The elimination of gender role stereotypes means that couples are free to establish the most satisfying relationship they can.
- The movement toward gender equality has also caused some losses, especially to women.

Key Terms
1. Culturally assigned behaviors assigned to a particular gender are called _gender roles_.
2. Fair distribution of responsibilities and duties is called _role equity_.
3. When one possess both male and female qualities, they are called _androgynous_.
4. _Norms_ are accepted behaviors and beliefs prescribed by a culture.
5. Behaviors expected by society when one assumes a particular position are called _roles_.
6. Persons who are born with both male and female sexual organs are called _hermaphrodites_.
7. A person who beliefs s/he is psychologically the opposite gender is called a _transsexual_.
8. A _transvestite_ receives sexual pleasure from dressing in clothing of the opposite gender.
9. The _double standard_ allows males more freedom of sexual expression than females.
10. _Rehabilitative Alimony_ is where the husband provides financial help to an ex-wife so she can receive training in order to enter the work force.
11. Sexual intercourse with an underage female is called _Statutory rape._.

True-False Questions
1. __T__ When gender roles are strictly prescribed by society, people tend to feel safe and secure.
2. __T__ Sexual identity includes both physiologically prescribed sex behaviors as well as socially prescribed gender behaviors.
3. __F__ Fertilized eggs can be identified as male or female within two days after conception.
4. __T__ Individuals learn masculine and feminine behavior from society; therefore, they can be changed.
5. __T__ In today's society, women are encouraged to seek careers outside the home but are made to feel guilty when they do not devote themselves fully to their families.
6. __F__ Although the women's movement changed women's lives, it did little to change the lives of men.
7. __T__ Stereotypic gender roles works well for couples who understand and freely accept this type of relationship.
8. __T__ Many women report that they resist being put into a stereotypic position by men yet they don't want to be referred to as feminists.
9. __F__ Over time American women have gained status and freedom in terms of sexuality, childbearing, and childrearing.
10. __F__ Sameness between the sexes, not equity, is the goal for males and females.

Multiple-Choice Questions

1. Increased freedom to choose fulfilling and equitable individual roles within intimate relationships
    a. will only hurt the relationship
    b. should lead to increased personal satisfaction and more fulfilling relationships
    c. will cause confusion as to who is responsible for what aspects of family life
    d. none of the above

2. Which is not one of the factors that determines gender identity?
    a. genetics
    b. hormone secretion that produces physical differences
    c. androgyny
    d. society's definition of gender roles

3. When someone is born with both male and female sexual organs, they are called a
    a. transsexual
    b. transvestite
    c. hermalee
    d. hermaphrodite

4. In Money and Ehrhardt's study of a twin whose gender was reassigned at birth, they found
    a. she developed role expectations that are culturally assigned.
    b. identity confusion on the part of the child.
    c. when the child was older, her true inclinations emerged.
    d. none of the above

5. In Ullian's theory of gender role development, the stage where there is a growing awareness that masculine and feminine traits can exist independently from biological features is
    a. stage three
    b. stage four
    c. stage one
    d. stage two

6. In Ullian's theory of gender role development, the stage where societal orientations are seen as fixed is
    a. stage one
    b. stage two
    c. stage three
    d. stage four

7. Research on sex role differences indicates that men have all of the following but one.
   a. math skills
   b. depth perception
   c. spatial skills
   d. night vision

8. Research on sex role differences indicates that women have all of the following but one.
   a. less tolerance to sound
   b. less sensitivity to heat
   c. manual dexterity
   d. verbal skills

9. The main reason why traditional roles for women have been found in almost all cultures is
   a. women don't have the physical strength men do
   b. religious teachings
   c. they bear children
   d. they are more emotional

10. Aggressiveness, self-confidence, and adventurousness are defined as being
   a. instrumental
   b. expressive
   c. androgynous
   d. traditional

11. Which statement is not true about gender roles?
   a. perceived advantages of one sex are the disadvantages of the other
   b. females complain about what they can't do, males about what they must do
   c. as more women choose nontraditional occupational roles, stereotypes tend to be reduced
   d. eventually society will completely do away with stereotypic roles

12. Which statement is not true about working class families?
   a. wife's working broadens her world and opens choices to her
   b. working wives often express job satisfaction while their husbands no not
   c. working class husbands like it when their wives work because they add to the family income
   d. working class husbands and wives express job satisfaction

13. Families with a female head of the house represent _____ of all poor families.
    a. one-fourth
    b. over one-half
    c. one-third
    d. over three-fourths

14. Role equity in a relationship means
    a. both men and women fulfill traditional gender roles
    b. traditional gender roles are mixed
    c. reversing traditional gender roles
    d. all of the above

15. How one views one's self is referred to as
    a. gender identity
    b. gender roles
    c. androgyny
    d. gender assignment

16. Sex of a child is determined by
    a. the woman's chromosomes
    b. hormone production
    c. the male's chromosome
    d. none of the above

17. A person who gains sexual pleasure from dressing like the opposite sex is called a
    a. hermaphrodite
    b. transvestite
    c. transsexual
    d. homosexual

18. In Ullian's theory of gender role development, the stage where an awareness that masculinity and
    femininity may exist independently from conformity to traditional roles and behavior is
    a. stage three
    b. stage one
    c. stage four
    d. stage two

19. The number of women having their first child after the age of thirty has _____ in the last sixteen years.
    a. doubled
    b. tripled
    c. stayed the same
    d. quadrupled

20. Which of the following statements is true about discrimination laws?
    a. few laws have been passed that deal with inequities in the work place
    b. the US has passed all the laws it needs, it only needs to enforce them
    c. although the sexes are more equal under the law, new inequities have emerged
    d. none of the above

21. Which of the following statements is false about women and men?
    a. men suffer more stress related illnesses than women
    b. more men attend and graduate from college than women
    c. although referred to as a minority, women outnumber men
    d. historically, approximately as many wives kill their husbands as visa versa

22. Two important stumbling blocks to liberation caused by stereotypical gender roles are
    a. economic deprivation of women and laws that discriminate against women
    b. prevailing stereotypic attitudes and economic deprivation of women
    c. women who do not work outside the home and laws that discriminate against women
    d. prevailing stereotypic attitudes and women that do not work outside the home

23. Which of the following is seen as a negative character trait of women?
    a. warm
    b. subjective
    c. social
    d. communicative

24. Which of the following is seen as a negative trait of men?
    a. aggressive
    b. adventurous
    c. unemotional
    d. decisive

25. Which is not one of the gains women have made in the past thirty years?
    a. flexible work schedules
    b. school sports
    c. maternity and paternal leaves
    d. equal pay

Critical Thinking and Decision Making
1. What are some advantages and disadvantages of traditional gender role attitudes?
2. How has the women's movement changed things for females as well as males?
3. How well do you handle stress? Do you become physically ill under enormous stress?
4. In your past and present relationships, have you shared tasks equally? Why or why not?
5. If you could create one law dealing with equality of men and women, what would it be?

Examining International Families
1. What are the pros and cons to holding the gender role attitudes of the Dani for men and women?
2. Compare and contrast the Dani with colonial America. Are they similar or different?

Debate the Issues
1. Do you think one parent should stay home to raise their children? Why?
2. If a parent should stay home to raise a child, how long should s/he do this? Is there an acceptable time to enter the labor force?
3. Should it be the mother or the father that stays home with the children?
4. What are single parents to do in raising children if they have no other choices - work outside the home or go on welfare?

Answers

Key Terms: 1   gender roles
              2   role equity
              3   androgynous
              4   norms
              5   roles
              6   hermaphrodites
              7   transsexual
              8   transvestite
              9   double standard
              10   rehabilitative alimony
              11   statutory rape

True/False: 1 T; 2 T; 3 F; 4 T; 5 T; 6 F; 7 T; 8 T; 9 F; 10 F

Multiple Choice: 1 b; 2 c; 3 d; 4 a; 5 c; 6 b; 7 d; 8 b; 9 c; 10 a; 11 d; 12 c; 13 b; 14 d; 15 a; 16 c; 17 b; 18 a; 19 d; 20 c; 21 b; 22 a; 23 b; 24 c; 25 d

Chapter 8
The Dual Worker Family: The Real American Family Revolution

Chapter Outline

- By 1992, 60 percent of all married-couple families were dual-earner families compared to 43 percent in 1967.

Women and the Economy
- Role equity has been restrained because the differential earning power of the sexes lock them into many traditional roles.
- More married women work outside the home today because:

  _____the economic need/to make ends meet_____ is the major reason.

  Real wages have increased dramatically.

  The number and kinds of jobs open to women have increased tremendously.

  Declining birthrates have reduced the demands of family work.

  Better education has opened job opportunities.

  Attitudes about the role of the woman in the family have changed greatly during this century.

  As the lower birthrate leads to reduced number of workers, women will become more and more important to maintain a sufficient work force.

Job Opportunities for Women
- The vast majority of women in the labor force are more concerned with general nondiscrimatory job availability and good pay than with obtaining _top management positions_ .
- Most women still work in the jobs and occupations that have historically been open to them.
- It was not until 1980 that women earned as many bachelor's degrees as men.

Pay Differentials Between Men and Women

- The gap between men's and women's average earnings has narrowed from 1955 to 1993 with the average women's earnings now at _____ percent of the average men's earnings.
- Research findings on reasons for the gap are mixed. Some argue the family and housekeeping duties frequently lead women to make different occupational choices than men; thus, women work fewer hours, accumulate less experience, and devote less time in acquiring skills. Others argue that discrimination makes it harder for women to find full-time work, to gain opportunities for training and advancement, or are in "male" occupations.
- Shaw and Shapiro found that earnings for women who had consistently made plans to work from the time they were in school were nearly __36__ percent higher than those who had never planned to work.
- _____ means that dissimilar jobs may be compared on the amount of training, effort, and skill; on the extent of similar responsibilities; and on the environment having an impact on the worker.
- Women in the youngest age groups earn considerably more compared to men than the overall average for women, suggesting that the pay differential will diminish with time.
- The unemployment gap between men and women has diminished over time and actually reversed in 1982. In 1993, the unemployment rate for women was 6.5 percent and for men was 7.1 percent.
- Between the mid-1960s and the mid-1990s, the percentage of wives earning more than their husbands increased from _____ to _____ percent.

Making the Decision to Become a Two-Earner Family: The Wife Goes to Work

- A woman must choose from four major work patterns:
  Pattern A: She works a few years before marriage then settles into the homemaker role for the rest of her life.
  Pattern B: She follows the same career pattern as men.
  Pattern C: She works until she has children, then stays home for a certain amount of time, and returns to the labor force.
  Pattern D: She stays in the labor force continuously with short time-outs to have children.
- Women most likely to follow Pattern _____ are women without children, African-American women, and women in professional and managerial jobs.
- Patterns _____ and _____ are limited by the job opportunities available.
- Increasingly, women are choosing Pattern _____ so their skills do not become outdated.
- In addition to the direct economic advantage of having another wage earner in the family, the working wife may derive greater satisfaction from her work, may feel more stimulated and fulfilled, and may enjoy higher self-esteem.
- Greater independence may postpone or effectively end the marriages of some women.

The Working Wife's Economic Contribution to the Family

- The costs of child care, transportation, taxes, social security, the need for more partially prepared and therefore more expensive foods, the need to send more clothing to the laundry, and the cost of new clothes to wear to work will reduce the impact of a second income.
- Full-time working wives increase family income by _____ percent in low-income families but only about _____ percent in middle-income families.

Household Activities and Supermothers

- To date, although men are doing more to offset the household pressures created by women's increased participation in the labor force, they still do not carry their fair share of household and child care work when their wives work.
- Hochschild discovered that married working women worked roughly _____ hours longer a week than men (paid work plus housework and child care).
- Studies have shown that husbands and fathers have not picked up the working wives' overload, and working wives and mothers indicate they do not have enough time for themselves.
- If a husband shares the family work, then he too may feel overburdened. If he does not, he may feel guilty about the wife's unfair work load.
- Thus, the revolution of the woman entering the paid labor force has not been accompanied by a revolution in how family work is handled, and the gap is causing family problems.

Deciding in Favor of Part-Time Work

- About _____ percent of working mothers with preschool children combine employment and caregiving by working part-time. Part-time work generally pays only _____ percent as much as full-time work.
- The _____ for part-time work means some people may opt for welfare because free medical care is available.
- Ninety percent of part-time employment occurs in the _____ industries.
- The number of women working part-time has dropped because more and more women seek full-time work.

Child Care and Parental Leave

- Today only one in three mothers stays home and provides full-time care for her children.
- In recent years women have argued and worked for family leave legislation and for government funding of day-care centers. In 1993, the first comprehensive federal family leave bill was passed that grants workers in companies with 50 or more workers 23 weeks unpaid leave for family emergencies including maternity leaves, elder care, and child-care leave. An equivalent job would be guaranteed upon returning from the leave.
- Traditionally, only a small minority of women with children under age six have been employed because of two reasons: _____ and_____ .

- The actual effects of substitute child care are difficult to determine. Parcel and Menaghan list many factors that influence the affect a working mother will have on her children: type of child care; family characteristics; number of children; dual career family or not; parental pay; work hours; type of job; child or children's characteristics; reasons for mother going to work; and acceptance of mother's working by family members.
- Substitute child-care cannot be wholly praised or condemned but must be judged on its specific merits.

Employers, Pregnant Employees, and Working Mothers
- Organizing the workplace so that a company can both successfully compete and provide personal growth for its employees and their families is a major challenge facing American employers.
- Better leave policies, more flexible working hours, job sharing, on-site child-care facilities, increased use of the home as a workplace, and job sharing are all possible ways to improve the relationship between family and work.

Marital Satisfaction in the Two-Earner Family
- The family may gain satisfaction through the wife's economic contribution; the family may lose satisfaction because she is no longer able to supply all of the caring and services of a full-time wife and mother.
- Research evidence on marital satisfaction when the wife works is mixed. Couples tend to score higher on marital satisfaction measures where the wife works from choice rather than economic necessity, in which the husband views the wife's employment favorably, where the wife works part-time, and in which equitable levels of power and influence occur.
- Husband's tend to be _____(more or less) satisfied than wives when both work.
- Happiness is more closely linked with congruence between the role expectations of the spouses rather than to any particular pattern of roles.
- Dual-career families tend to produce children whose attitudes are more egalitarian and who prefer dual-career families themselves.
- Daughters of working mothers tend to view women as more competent and view female employment as less threatening to marriage than daughters of nonworking mothers.

Work and Family: Sources of Conflict
- Traditionally, a husband's family usually must bend to his work demands; a wife's work must usually bend to her family's demands.
- The dual-worker family with children suffers the most from lack of time, especially parenting time. Some estimates indicate the amount of time parents have with their children has dropped _____ % since 1965.
- Continuing restructuring and downsizing by business not only causes unemployment but also increased job insecurity for those still employed.
- Husband's tend to view relocation experiences _____ (more or less) favorably than their wives.
- Specific patterns of role behavior on the job and in the family may be incompatible.

- About one million couples in the US have commuter marriages. Such couples tend to be free of childrearing responsibilities, to be older, to be married longer, to have established careers, to have higher educational levels, to have high-ranking occupations, and to have high income levels.

Summary
- Many consider the number of women entering the work force to be the major revolution affecting the American family in this century.
- Women still earn a disproportionately lower income than their male counterparts.
- Career opportunities are still narrower for women than for men.
- The working mother is often overburdened, performing the duties of her job as well as being the major worker in the home.
- Increasing job availability has made women more independent than they have been in the past.
- The lower incomes often received by women blunt some of the possible advantages of working.

Key Terms
1. A child who stays at home by himself/herself after school is called a __latch key child__.
2. When two dissimilar jobs require the same amount of training, effort, skill, and responsibility they are referred to as having __Comparable worth__.
3. The type of work pattern where a woman ceases to work in the labor force in order to marry and have children is called __Pattern A__.
4. When a woman stays in the labor force with short time-outs to have children, this is referred to as __Pattern D__ work type.
5. The type of work pattern for women that is the same as men is called __Pattern B__.
6. When women leave the labor force to have children, only to return several years later, it is referred to as __Pattern C__ work type.

True-False Questions
1. __T__ In the past, most women in the American labor force were single.
2. __T__ Women are America's best source of cheap labor.
3. __F__ The vast majority of women in the labor force are more concerned with obtaining top management positions than they are with nondiscriminatory job availability.
4. __F__ A woman who takes a break from the labor force to have children often earns more after she returns to the labor force.
5. __T__ Greater work availability is one factor in why women leave unsatisfying marriages.
6. __F__ Most women are in the labor force for self-fulfillment rather than economic necessity.
7. __F__ With women's increased participation in the labor force, men are now doing their fair share of household and child care work.

8. ___T___ When women contribute economically to the family, they obtain more power within the marital relationship.

9. ___F___ Dual career families tend to produce children who do not want dual career families when they marry because they focus on the negative aspects of the mother working outside the home.

10. ___F___ Past research on the dual-career family reported that the impact of dual career stress is felt mostly by men.

Multiple-Choice Questions

1. What percentage of mothers with children under six work or are looking for work?
   a. one-fourth
   b. ninety percent
   c. over one-half
   d. slightly over one-third

2. Which women are more likely to be year-round full-time workers?
   a. African-American
   b. Hispanic
   c. White
   d. Asian

3. The main reason the majority of wives work is
   a. self-fulfillment
   b. boredom at home
   c. declining birthrates
   d. economic necessity

4. Women now hold _____ of all managerial positions.
   a. one-fourth
   b. three-fourths
   c. almost one-half
   d. over one-half

5. The unintentional blocking of women from upper management positions is called
   a. discrimination
   b. the glass ceiling
   c. career blocking
   d. none of the above

6. Which of the following is why an earnings gap exists?
    a. discrimination against women
    b. better training for men
    c. men are primary breadwinners and therefore more committed to their work
    d. all of the above

7. When looking at women's earnings as a percentage of men's earnings by age, the results indicate
    a. older women earn more compared to men than the overall average for women
    b. younger women earn more compared to men than the overall average for women
    c. women earn as much as men do at any age
    d. middle age women earn more compared to men than the overall average for women

8. Of the four major work patterns, which type becomes the traditional family after the woman marries?
    a. pattern A
    b. pattern B
    c. pattern C
    d. pattern D

9. African-American women, women without children, and women in professional jobs are more likely to follow which work pattern for women?
    a. pattern A
    b. pattern B
    c. pattern C
    d. pattern D

10. Of the four major work patterns for women, which pattern is a woman in when she remains in the labor force continuously with short time-outs to have children?
    a. pattern A
    b. pattern B
    c. pattern C
    d. pattern D

11. Increasing work availability for women has caused which of the following?
    a. increased freedom within marriage
    b. increased freedom from marriage
    c. freedom to seek new roles
    d. all of the above

12. The average age of marriage for men and women is
      a. 23 and 20
      b. 24.5 and 23.5
      c. 26.5 and 24.5
      d. 25 for both

13. Besides economic advantages, another benefit for working women is
      a. sharing equal power with her husband
      b. personal satisfaction
      c. being able to hire domestic help
      d. none of the above

14. What is the single biggest expense of a working mother with young children?
      a. child care
      b. professional clothing
      c. the cost of commuting to and from work
      d. continued education in order to retain the job

15. Hochschild analyzed family time distribution studies and found that married working mothers work
      a. 20 more hours per week than men.
      b. 10 more hours per week than men.
      c. 15 more hours per week than men.
      d. 35 more hours per week than men.

16. The effects of working on women is
      a. role overload and strain
      b. decrease in leisure time
      c. quality of household work declines
      d. all of the above

17. For the working woman, _____ is the most precious commodity.
      a. money
      b. more leisure time
      c. more time with family
      d. none of the above

18. What are the two greatest strains placed on the family when both spouses work?
    a. finding child care and long hours on the job
    b. lack of time with family and long hours on the job
    c. lack of time with family and keeping up with household duties
    d. child care and keeping up with household duties

19. Verbrugge and Madans found _____ was the strongest and most consistent predictor of a women's good health.
    a. employment
    b. marriage
    c. parenthood
    d. support network

20. Which two factors have worked to keep mothers of young children out of the labor force?
    a. child care arrangements and money
    b. work hours and domestic responsibilities
    c. low wages and child care arrangements
    d. child care arrangements and societal attitudes about mothers and young children

21. If the family is to survive both parents working, and businesses are to have satisfied, productive workers, the American society needs to
    a. increase wages
    b. integrate obligations of both family and work
    c. provide more and better child care
    d. reorganize the workplace

22. Which is not one of the benefits companies experience when they provide child care for their employees?
    a. lower employee turnover
    b. lower absenteeism
    c. less tardiness
    d. fewer recruitment problems

23. Which family seems to have more adjustment problems when the wife goes to work?
    a. lower class
    b. middle class
    c. upper class
    d. poverty

24. Studies indicate that American parents believe that _____ is the most important cause of the fragmentation and stress in family life.
    a. both parents working
    b. spending less time with their families
    c. wanting more for their children than what they had as children
    d. the stress that accompanies economic conditions

25. Which of the following is not a characteristic of commuter marriages?
    a. established careers
    b. long marriages
    c. high educational levels
    d. young children

Critical Thinking and Decision Making
1. Should women drop out of the labor force when their children are very young? Why?
2. What do you think is the main cause of the break down of the American family?
3. Do you think women will attain equal status with men in the work place in terms of wages and respect for their jobs? Why?
4. What are the advantages and disadvantages of each of the four work patterns of women?
5. Would society change its views toward work and families if more men fit into each of the work patterns for women? How?
6. Identify solutions that will help men and women equally share work, child care, and household tasks.
7. Identify the advantages and disadvantages of working part-time as opposed to full-time.

Answers

Key Terms: 1   latch key child
               2   comparable worth
               3   pattern A
               4   pattern D
               5   pattern B
               6   pattern C

True/False: 1 T; 2 T; 3 F; 4 F; 5 T; 6 F; 7 F; 8 T; 9 F; 10 F

Multiple Choice: 1 c; 2 a; 3 d; 4 c; 5 b; 6 d; 7 b; 8 a; 9 b; 10 d; 11 d; 12 c; 13 b; 14 a; 15 c; 16 d; 17 c; 18 b; 19 a; 20 d; 21 b; 22 c; 23 a; 24 b; 25 d

Chapter 9
The Importance of Making Sound Economic Decisions

Chapter Outline

- Work, money, and intimacy are closely intertwined for most families.
- While most courting couples do not discuss each other's financial values, money matters are the topics most commonly discussed, and money is the most common source of conflict for America's married couples.
- Economic stability and security is necessary for the development of family strength.
- In 1993, the average full-time earnings of a college graduate exceed the average for high school graduates by $24,000 for men and $_____ for women.
- Married couples earnings are more than twice that of female householders with no husband present.
- About _____ percent of all American households owe money at some time in each year.
- Knowing how to budget, spend, save, borrow, and invest are important skills for personal and family stability and happiness.

<u>Slowly Drowning in a Sea of Debt</u>
- Marriage usually means a drastic reduction in the standard of living for most young couples since they have probably shared their parents' standard of living.
- Many young Americans, especially men, are infatuated with automobiles. The cost of car ownership is higher than most realize: e.g. a new Ford Escort costs 33 cents per mile to operate. The value of an automobile _____ with time.
- Most families that go bankrupt are lower- and middle-class families who slowly become overburdened with increasing debts. _____ percent of those who file bankruptcy use credit and are in debt trouble again within five years.

- Signs that you are headed for bankruptcy: _____ , _____ ,
no plans for retirement, many credit cards with considerable balances, assets are not liquid, can not resist
buying something you want, and thinking financial problems will take care of themselves.

Making Good Credit, Borrowing, and Installment Buying Decisions
- Credit and debt are directly opposed to personal _____ .
- People borrow for two basic reasons: to buy consumer goods and services and to invest in tangible
assets.
- Discount interest is usually charged for consumer debt such as cars, furniture, and clothes. It is higher
than investment debt which is used for tangible assets, such as real estate or businesses.
- Simple interest is usually charged for investment debt. It is only paid on the unpaid balance of the loan.

Discount Interest: Consumer Purchases
- On a discount interest loan, one pays interest on the full amount of the loan each year even though you
have paid back part of the loan. A simple way to calculate the approximate interest rate on such a loan is
to _____ the stated interest rate.
- Credit card interest rates usually range from 17 to 21 percent. If used properly, a credit card can give
you thirty days of interest free credit if you pay it off within a month.
- By 1993, 32 percent of high-school seniors and 82 percent of college students had at least one credit
card. The average American has _____ credit cards with a total balance of $2800.

Simple Interest: Home Loans
- Simple interest is charged when borrowing to buy tangible assets such as a home. Monthly payments are
the same over the term of the loan, and each month you will pay less interest and more against the
principal.
- _____ : the amount of money borrowed.
- _____ : the charge, usually stated as a percentage of the principal, that is paid for borrowing.

Financial Problems and Marital Strain
- Financial difficulties affect all areas of a relationship, not just the economic realm.

The Seductive Society: Credit and Advertising
- Thrift and saving are no longer considered virtues and have been replaced with _____ and _____ .
- Spending is important in a credit-oriented inflationary society. Financial reports often state: "strong
growth in consumption reflects rising income and bodes well for the economy." Such attitudes
encourage spending.
- Galbraith observes that two broad propositions undergird consumer demand in America:
    The _____ does not diminish appreciably as more of them are satisfied.
    Wants originate in the _____ of the consumer and are capable of _____ .

- Economic contentment appears to be more closely related to one's attitude and values than to one's actual economic level.
- Advertising sometimes manipulates the consumer into buying regardless of the consequence.
- Packard questions the morality of advertising aimed at the following: encouraging housewives to be irrational and impulsive in buying family food; manipulating small children; playing on hidden weakness and frailties such as anxieties, aggressive feelings, dread of conformity, and infantile hangovers; and developing public attitudes of wastefulness toward natural resources.

Effective Money Management
- Financial matters are the most widely reported causes of family discord. Almost _____ percent of young couples who divorce by age thirty report that financial problems were a primary cause of the divorce.
- Monetary decisions can be handled in six ways:

  _____ .

  _____ .

  The couple makes decisions jointly.
  One spouse controls the income but gives the other an allowance.
  Each spouse has separate funds, and the couple shares agreed-on financial obligations.
  The couple has a joint bank account on which each can draw as necessary.

To Pool or Not to Pool Family Money?
- Couples who pool their money seem neither more nor less satisfied with their money management.
- Decisions about pooling influences decisions about who is responsible for spending the funds and is related to power and control within the relationship.
- Generally, the partner who provides the primary monetary support also claims most of the power in the relationship.
- Power through monetary control is greatest in the single-earner family.
- No evidence suggests that a particular manner of monetary allocation is most desirable----most important is that partners agree and are comfortable with the manner of allocation chosen.

Budgeting: Enlightened Control of Spending
- A _____ is a plan of spending.
- Housing, food, and taxes make up over _____ percent of the annual expenses for a four-person, medium-income family.
- Budgeting and long-term monetary planning lead to financial independence---the freedom to do what you want.

Saving Through Wise Spending

- Wise spending is another way of _____ . Buying when an item is "on sale", seeking out bargains, buying used instead of new, being aware of consumer traps in marketing, and studying seasonal fluctuations in order to buy at the right time are all ways to spend more wisely.
- One should do extensive research before buying "big ticket" items.
- Various consumer traps include _____ , _____ , _____ , telemarketing, winning contests, free goods, off brand items, hard sell, home repairs, magazines, credit repair, free travel, and advance fee loans.

The Economy and the African American, Latino, and Asian American Family

- In 1993:
  The median family incomes from highest to lowest were: White, Asian American, Black, and Hispanic.
  The unemployment rates from lowest to highest were: Asian American, White, Hispanic, and Black.
  Poverty rates ranged from lowest to highest: White, Hispanic, and African American.
  In all cases, higher monthly incomes correlated with higher educational achievement.
- Those groups with the highest percentages of both women and men graduating from high school tend to be the groups with the lowest percentage below the poverty level.
- Families with a female head of house and no husband present account for _____ of all poor families.
- The large proportion of African American families below the poverty line tends to be the result of the large number of single-parent families in the African American population. However, over _____ of African American families have an annual income above the national median.

Inflation and Recession

- Since World War II, inflation has generally averaged 4 to 6 percent per year.
- _____ costs are the absolute prices for items.
- The Consumer Price Index (CPI) is calculated on a fixed market basket of goods and services measured in 91 urban areas across the country.
- Nominal costs can decrease in recessions and depressions or with technological breakthroughs that lower production costs. However, nominal costs generally _____ with inflation.
  Techniques to combat inflation: _____ .
  Select high-yield savings accounts whenever possible.
  Try to include a cost-of-living clause in employment contracts.
  Try not to let inflation panic you into buying before you are ready.
  Learn about investments.
  Understand that inflation tends to favor the borrower.
  Try to buy wisely.
  Have more members of the family work.
  Conserve and save to accumulate investment funds.

- Most likely inflation will occur _____ (more or less) frequently than recession.
- Techniques to protect against recession:

  _____ .

  Beware of investments with a large balloon payment due in the near future.
  If recession is foreseen, try to maintain a larger percentage of your assets in cash.
  Make sure that your financial position is flexible.

Deciding What Insurance Is Needed

- Every family must have _____ , automobile insurance if they own a car, and

  _____ .

- Medical insurance is an absolute necessity because medical cost have become so high.
- Automobile insurance is essential, and many states require it.
- Fire insurance is mandatory when obtaining a mortgage.
- Life insurance is not absolutely necessary; however, it can protect against premature death and long tern disability.
- The two types of life insurance are _____ and _____ .
- _____ insurance is less expensive for the same coverage because it accumulates no savings.
  Enough life insurance should be purchased to cover death costs, taxes, outstanding debts, and enable the family to continue functioning. This will depend on the individual family.

Deciding to Buy a Home

- About 65 percent of families own homes in the US. It often is a major source of savings for retired people.
- Home ownership represents a dream for many young couples. Two factors may argue against home ownership: _____ and _____ .
- Five major considerations in buying a home: _____ , _____ , size, livability, and status.

The Decision to Invest

- Investments range from very conservative bank savings accounts to highly speculative gambles.
- A positive attitude toward investment is actually more important than the investment itself.
- Investing $100 a month for 40 years earning 12 percent will accumulate $1 million.
- Investment involves these steps: _____ , _____ , and _____ .

Gaining Freedom Through Investment

- Forbes, Fortune, Business Week, and Money are magazines from which one can learn about investing.
- The Depository Institutions Deregulation Act of 1980 opened the way for checking accounts that earn interest, higher interest on savings accounts, and a variety of investment vehicles for the small investor.

- Once a savings account has been accumulated, one can begin to investigate a broader range of investments.
- _____ mortgages involve loaning money with real estate as security for the debt. They require considerable money which is tied up for a long time.
- _____ involve loaning money with real estate as security after a first mortgage has already been placed against the property. They are held usually for a few years only, are usually for considerably lesser amounts than the first mortgage, and generally yield higher interest rates.
- A _____ is a group of investors that form a partnership to make an investment, usually to buy real estate or a business.
- Apartments and commercial rental properties require time as well as money since the properties must be managed.
- _____ are businesses that are supported by a large company's reputation, experience, backing, and advertising and require the owner to use the parent company's products and maintain a given standard of service.
- Land speculation and commodities are gambles that future values of land or commodities such as farm products or raw materials will be worth more than the current purchase price. They should be avoided by the small investor because of the risk.
- Oil, mining, and invention backing are even more speculative than land speculation and commodities.
- Stocks and bonds offer a variety of means for investments both large and small.
- _____ are promissory notes companies issue to raise funds. They are usually issued in multiples of a thousand dollars, pay a specified, usually low interest for a specific amount of time, usually involve a low risk, and can be redeemed for the face amount at the end of its term.
- _____ give the owner the right to a portion of the assets of the company issuing the stock. They are issued to raise money for the company, usually for expansion, allow the owner to vote at stockholders' meetings, and are usually listed on stock exchanges.
- _____ are shares of a large, diversified group of stocks and bonds.

Summary
- The family is the major unit of consumption in the U. S.
- Buying consumer goods on credit can lock a person into an inflexible life pattern.
- A thorough understanding of credit, installment buying, interest costs, and budgeting can work to a family's benefit.
- The day-to-day handling of money can be a problem if family partners have different values about money.
- Inflation is the primary economic enemy of the newly married couple.
- Insurance should be considered a necessity.
- The American dream of home ownership for every family may be fading in the face of increased housing prices.
- Investments are a means of supplementing income and making money work to produce more money.
- Investments can be plotted along a continuum from low risk, low return to high risk, high return.

Key Terms

1. Interest that is charged on the total amount of the loan for the entire loan period is called

    _____.

2. Interest that is charged only on the unpaid balance of the loan is called

    _____.

3. A plan of spending to assure basic needs are met and some desires are obtained is called a

    _____.

4. A absolute price for an item is called the _____.

True-False Questions

1. _____ Financial worries and marginal economic survival lower personal and marital satisfaction.
2. _____ Economic contentment of an individual appears to be more closely related to one's attitudes and values than to one's actual economic level.
3. _____ Personal freedom and indebtedness are inversely related; the more debt you assume, the less personal freedom you have.
4. _____ Only a small minority of young couples who divorce by age thirty report financial problems as a primary cause of divorce.
5. _____ An important step in effective money management is to determine ahead of time how most monetary decisions will be made.
6. _____ Families with a female head of house and no husband present account for one-fourth of all poor families.
7. _____ The best insurance protection for the least amount of money is whole life insurance.
8. _____ Credit use in the United States has allowed Americans to maintain the world's highest standard of living.
9. _____ If the money spent on home ownership was saved and invested wisely, it would probably make more money than would accrue through appreciation of a home.
10. _____ As long as a family stays healthy, in economically hard times, they can do without health insurance.

Multiple-Choice Questions

1. What percentage of wives are in the labor force?
    a. one-fourth
    b. three-fourths
    c. one-half
    d. two-thirds

2. Which statement is correct about economic success and family success?
     a. economic success guarantees family success
     b. economic failure almost always leads to family problems and breakdown
     c. there is no relationship between the two
     d. the threat of economic failure brings the family together

3. What is the most common source of conflict for American families?
     a. money
     b. whether they should buy a house
     c. in-laws
     d. investment opportunities

4. Which is one of the first things threatened by unemployment?
     a. the family's perception of the unemployed member
     b. self-esteem
     c. personal identity
     d. loss of family

5. The modern American family is the basic economic unit of society because
     a. they are a production unit
     b. they are a consuming unit
     c. they are a production and consuming unit on an equal basis
     d. they have a large amount of debt

6. _____ is/are one of the few products in the inflationary economy that usually declines in
   value.
     a. land
     b. houses
     c. jewelry
     d. automobiles

7. Of those who file for bankruptcy, what percent use credit and are in debt trouble again within five years?
     a. twenty-five
     b. fifty
     c. eighty
     d. ninety

8. Which statement is true about credit buying in the United States?
    a. credit has given the means for a more fulfilling life, but its has also enslaved many
       people at great psychological costs
    b. credit is the downfall of the American family
    c. the use of credit has given individuals more personal freedom
    d. all of the above

9. People borrow for two reasons, they are
    a. to invest and to purchase a home
    b. to consolidate debts and survive form month to month
    c. to buy goods and services and to purchase a home
    d. to buy goods and services and to invest in tangible assets

10. Which type of interest is charged only on the unpaid balance of the loan?
    a. simple interest
    b. discount interest
    c. compound interest
    d. none of the above

11. What is the fastest growing component of overall consumer debt?
    a. home mortgages
    b. car loans
    c. credit cards
    d. none of the above

12. What percentage of all full-time four-year college students have and use credit?
    a. one-fourth
    b. three-fourths
    c. two-thirds
    d. one-half

13. Experts suggest that payments for debt should total no more than _____ of spendable income.
    a. 40 %
    b. 20 %
    c. 30 %
    d. 50 %

14. Which statement best describes the relationship between money and power?
    a. regardless of how much money he makes, the husband has the most power
    b. women have more power than men if she works outside the home
    c. generally, the partner who makes the most money has the most power
    d. there is no relationship between money and power in marital relationships

15. Which statement best describes the way couples should handle money?
    a. couples should pool their money and have a joint account
    b. couples should keep their money separate
    c. the one who makes the most money should have the most control
    d. no method is most desirable; partners should agree and be comfortable with the chosen method

16. A consumer trap where a store advertises one product and then claims to be out of the product when one goes to purchase it is called
    a. bait and switch
    b. low ball
    c. high ball
    d. off brand items

17. A consumer trap where businesses offer free extras but make the customer pay a higher price for the other goods is called
    a. high ball
    b. free goods
    c. hard sell
    d. bait and switch

18. The value of consumer goods already purchased usually:
    a. increases in value over time
    b. is about the same as time passes
    c. decreases in value over time
    d. none of the above

19. Which is not one of the ways that families can combat inflation?
    a. remember that inflation tends to favor the agency lending the money
    b. have more family members work
    c. minimize your cash holdings
    d. select high yield savings accounts

20. Which of the following investments is considered the most risky?
   a. franchises
   b. land speculations
   c. syndicates
   d. oil, mining, and invention backing

21. Which type of stock market investment is considered low risk?
   a. common blue chip stock
   b. bonds
   c. mutual funds
   d. preferred stock

22. When a group of individuals form a partnership and raise money for investment purposes, it is called a
   a. franchise
   b. corporation
   c. syndicate
   d. none of the above

23. A form of IOU or promissory note that companies issue when they need funds is called
   a. bonds
   b. preferred stock
   c. common stock
   d. mutual funds

24. _____ is the primary economic enemy of the newly married couple.
   a. insurance
   b. debt
   c. inflation
   d. none of the above

25. Stocks that are really shares of large blocks of other stocks are called
   a. common stocks
   b. mutual funds
   c. common stock
   d. bonds

Critical Thinking and Decision Making

1. Identify the positive and negative effects of advertising.
2. When is using credit helpful? When is it harmful?
3. What have you purchased, or someone has purchased for you, that primarily met your need to "have what others have" or to impress others?
4. Would you pool your income with your spouse's? Why or why not? Who would pay what bills?
5. What would be the characteristics of an automobile that you would purchase? Why?

Examining International Families

1. If the economy of Mexico is improving, what is the incentive to stay in Mexico if the per capita income is greater in the US?
2. Mexicans place greater importance on the extended family than do Americans. Will this importance diminish as more Mexicans achieve the middle-class? Why or why not?

Debate the Issues

What percentage of your take-home pay is used to pay credit cards?

Answers

Key Terms: 1   discount interest
               2   simple interest
               3   budget
               4   nominal costs

True/False: 1 T; 2 T; 3 T; 4 F; 5 T; 6 F; 7 F; 8 T; 9 T; 10 F

Multiple Choice: 1 c; 2 b; 3 a; 4 b; 5 b; 6 d; 7 c; 8 a; 9 d; 10 a; 11 c; 12 d; 13 b; 14 c; 15 d; 16 a; 17 b; 18 c; 19 a; 20 d; 21 b; 22 c; 23 a; 24 c; 25 b

Chapter 10
Human Sexuality

Chapter Outline

- Sex is many things: the foundation for human intimate relationships, the basis of family procreation, communication and closeness, and the source of pleasure.

Human Sexuality Compared With Other Species
- For lower animals, sex is controlled by built-in biological mechanisms.
- Human beings have no biologically built-in mechanisms, so sexuality is learned, and different societies teach different things about sexuality.
- Sex for human females differs from that of other animals: females are capable of intense orgasmic response, and females are not necessarily more responsive during ovulation.
- Compared to other species, human sexuality is: pervasive, involving humans psychologically as well as physiologically; under conscious control; affected by learning and social factors; largely directed at an individual's beliefs and attitudes; less directly attached to reproduction; able to serve other purposes such as pair bonding and communication; and more a source of pleasure.

Human Sexuality
- Over the past thirty years, sexual attitudes and behaviors for American society have become freer, more diverse, and more open to public view.
- The _____ that promoted sex for men and discouraged it for women has broken down.
- One of the revolutionary changes affecting the family and intimate relationships has been the better understanding and acceptance by women of their sexuality.
- Sexual freedom brings with it _____ (more or less) responsibility for one's actions.

A New Sexual Revolution?
- While sexual attitudes and practices have been liberalized, factors that have modified the changes brought about by freer sexual freedom are the epidemic return of sexually transmitted diseases, the fact that recreational sex alone becomes dull and boring, the fact that many women indicate they feel less fulfilled with sexual liberation because affection, tenderness, and cuddling is more important to their happiness than sex, and the practical outcome of more sex is more children.
- A Psychology Today survey indicated that _____ percent of men and _____ percent of women believe sex without love is either unenjoyable or unacceptable. Twenty-five years ago, 66 percent of respondents indicated they would not have sex with someone they didn't love.
- Commitment, caring, and the broader aspects of meaningful intimate relationships seem to have been lost with sexual liberation.

Differences Between Male and Female Sexuality
- Young girls develop an interest in sex earlier than boys since puberty begins about two years earlier for girls on the average. Then, boys' interest soars above that of girls until the age of about 30. Men's interest remains relatively constant throughout adulthood, while women's interest peaks in their thirties or forties.
- Based on sex drive alone, _____ men and younger women and older women and younger men make the most compatible partners.
- _____ is sexually explicit material without emotional involvement.
- _____ is sexually explicit material that has emotional and romantic overtones of sensuality and caring.
- Men are more easily stimulated by pornography. Women react more positively to erotica.
- Masters, Johnson, and Kolodny found that both heterosexual males and females were aroused by fantasies of replacement sex partners, forced sex encounters, observations of sexual activity, and homosexual encounters.
- The capacity for orgasm differs more widely among individual women than among individual men. Women must learn how to reach orgasm.
- When multiple orgasms are experienced, women's pleasure generally rises with repeated orgasms; men's generally declines.
- Sexual desire for women tends to be cyclical and related to the menstrual cycle although patterns vary among women. There is no counterpart for men.
- _____ is a term applied to both physical and psychological symptoms experienced by women which are related to menstruation.

The Physiology of the Sexual Response

- Masters and Johnson identify four phases of sexual response: _____ , _____ , _____ , and _____ .
- Women are capable of repeating the four-phase cycle immediately after resolution. The male usually experiences a refractory period lasting from a few minutes to several hours before the cycle can be repeated.
- Females have a greater diversity of sensation and reaction to sexual stimulation during orgasm than males do.
- Levels of testosterone seem to influence women's level of desire just as it does men.
- Women can have multiple orgasms. It is not necessary to stimulate the clitoris directly for orgasm to occur, though such stimulation produces the quickest orgasm for most women.
- Masters and Johnson found that the myth that the female responds more slowly to stimulation is not necessarily true. The much-discussed slowness in arousal is probably due to cultural repression rather than some physiological difference.
- Simultaneous orgasm for partners is not necessary for complete sexual satisfaction.
- Many sexologists now consider masturbation an important and necessary part of sexual expression rather than a taboo behavior.

Does Sexual Addiction Exist?

- Sexual addiction involves the inability to control or stop sexual behaviors that lead to harmful consequences. Sexually addicted persons separate sex from love and caring.
- Some researchers believe sexual addiction is a problem for some Americans; others believe it is a myth.
- Researchers argue against the existence of addiction since culture defines acceptable behavior not biology and sex is the only type of addiction that is not given up as part of the treatment.
- _____ : casual sex with numerous partners.
- The acceptance of _____ , _____ , and sexual stimulation in children are all behaviors that are found in other cultures but are taboo in America.

Marital Sex: Can I Keep the Excitement Alive?

- Clements found that 67 percent of married couples expressed satisfaction with their sex lives compared to only _____ percent for single persons.
- Factors that diminish sexual interaction and excitement after marriage include: monetary concerns, job demands, household chores, and children.
- Husbands tend to complain _____ (more or less) than wives about children interfering with sex lives.
- Sex can serve as a bonding agent for married couples and improve the relationship.
- Inhibited sexual desire is a pervasive lack of interest in sex.
- There is no "normal" standard of frequency of sexual interaction for married couples. The only real standard is that both partners are happy and satisfied with their sexual interaction.
- As with other aspects of intimate relationships, married couples must work to maintain a fulfilling sex life.

Sex and the Aging Process

- Men and women who have been sexually active early in life tend to remain so even in their eighties and nineties, although frequency of intercourse may be limited by physical health and social circumstance.
- Michael found that 66 percent of men and _____ percent of women ages 50 to 59 had sex a few times or more a month.
- Masters and Johnson found three criteria for continuing sexual activity regardless of age: good general health, interesting and interested sexual partner, and the sexual organs must be used, particularly for males over 50 years of age.
- _____ is the cessation of the menstrual cycle in women. It generally occurs between the ages of forty-six and fifty-one.
- Men do not entirely lose their ability to reproduce as women do.
- _____ therapy is used to reduce the negative symptoms of menopause such as "hot flashes", excessive fatigue, dizziness, muscular aches and pains, and emotional upset.
- Estrogen also reduces the incidence of heart disease, prevents osteoporosis, reduces the incidence of colon cancer, and helps preserve skin elasticity.
- Negative side effects include suspected links to breast and ovarian cancer, the continuation of menstrual bleeding, and continuation of premenstrual symptoms.

Sex and Drugs

- _____ : a substance that arouses sexual desire. So far, no such substance has been found.
- Alcohol loosens control and inhibitions but may be detrimental to sexual performance.
- Marijuana may seem to increase sexual sensitivity, probably because it affects perception but it too may be detrimental to sexual performance.
- LSD, amphetamines, and cocaine can seriously destroy one's general health.
- _____ : substances that diminish sexual desire. Saltpeter has no known direct physiological effect on sexual behavior.
- Sedatives, antiandrogens, anticholenergic, and antiadrenergic drugs are drugs used for specific health problems that work to diminish sexual responses.
- Psychotropic drugs (tranquilizers), heroin, morphine, methadone, and nicotine generally impair sexual interest or activity.

Sexually Transmitted Diseases (STD)

- STDs remain a critical health problem with persons under age 25 accounting for the majority of cases.
- Three factors have played a role in the resurgence of STDs: the pill brought on a reduction in the use of condoms, antibiotics have lulled people into apathy, and the increased sexual activity among the young, particularly the increase in number of sexual partners.
- Women suffer more long-term consequences of STDs and are more likely to acquire an STD than their male partners.

- Genital _____ : a disease caused by a virus similar to the one that causes cold sores. Blisters occur on the genitals and contain a fluid that is extremely infectious. No known cure exists, and the virus remains in the body, possibly to reactivate later.
- Acquired Immune Deficiency Syndrome (AIDS): a disease caused by the human immunodeficiency virus (HIV) that damages the immune system. Persons usually die within one or two years of diagnosis from opportunistic diseases that strike because of the damaged immune system.
- Lymphocyte, or "lymph cells" are destroyed by the HIV. They produce antibodies that fight infection and are the basic cell in the body's immune system, the body's biological defense system against disease.
- Symptoms of AIDS include: loss of appetite, swollen glands, severe tiredness, unexplained persistent or recurrent fevers, persistent unexplained cough, persistent white coating or spots inside the mouth or throat, persistent purple or brown lumps or spots on the skin, and nervous system problems.
- Within a few weeks of exposure some HIV-infected persons develop an illness for one or two weeks. Tests for antibodies seldom become positive until six weeks to six months later. Months or years may pass without signs of AIDS in the infected person. Usually five to twelve years after initial exposure, the characteristic signs of AIDS appear. Some researchers predict an incubation period as long as 20 years is possible. Once AIDS appears, death usually follows within two years.
- _____ percent of all persons who have developed AIDS have died.
- _____ : having a virus present in the blood but showing no symptoms of the disease.
- Researchers estimate that 1.5 to 2 million persons in the US are AIDS seropositive.
- _____ percent of AIDS cases involve homosexual or bisexual men and twenty-five percent of cases involve present or past users of intravenous drugs.
- Eighty-six percent of AIDS cases in the US are found in men. Seventy-five percent of cases involve men twenty to fifty years of age. Twelve percent of case are found in women. The remaining 2 percent are found in children.
- Until now, AIDS has infected very specific groups in the US. Engaging indiscriminately in sexual and drug activities with multiple partners is particularly dangerous. AIDS is also spread from mothers to newborns during pregnancy and birth and through the mother's milk after birth. Occasionally, it is spread by transfusions of blood or blood products.
- HIV is primarily spread through the sharing of virus-infected lymphocytes in semen and in blood.
- _____ is the sexual behavior that is the best way to avoid being infected.
- Receptive anal-rectal intercourse appears to be the most dangerous sexual practice.
- Using condoms (safer sex) does not eliminate the danger completely.
- AIDS can be transmitted through vaginal intercourse, and females are more likely to be infected than males.
- Intravenous drug users who share syringes and needles are the second largest group of people with AIDS in the US, and appears to be the major bridge to infecting women and children.
- Since 1985, blood donations have been tested for contamination by HIV through a test called _____ . The CDC suggests the chances of infection by transfusion are about 1 in 60,000.

- Shaking hands, touching a friend, superficial kissing, drinking from the same cup, working in the same office, eating food served by infected persons, being sneezed or coughed on, and using public restrooms are not likely to spread AIDS. If it was possible, such spreading would be called _____ transmission.
- If a person is a carrier of the virus and has sexual relations with another, the carrier may be liable if the partner develops AIDS in the future.
- Clamydial infections are the most common bacterial STDs in the US and are the leading cause of preventable infertility and ectopic pregnancy.
- Other STDs include: pelvic inflammatory disease (PID), genital warts, gonorrhea, syphilis, and hepatitis B.

Summary
- Sexuality pervades the lives of humans.
- All human societies try to control sexual expression, but the controls vary from one society to another.
- In the US, sexual behavior has become freer since the 1960s.
- Males and females are physiologically similar, having developed their sexual organs from common structures, but they also differ in some respects.
- Both males and females share the same basic physical responses during sexual activity.
- Satisfactory sex at older ages is much more prevalent than many people believe.
- Unfortunately, sexually transmitted diseases too often accompany sexual activity.

Key Terms
1. Stimulation of the genital organs, by means other than intercourse is called _____.
2. The small organ at the upper end of the female genitals is called the _____.
3. The climax of excitement during sexual arousal is called an _____.
4. A pervasive and continuing disinterest in sex is referred to as an _____.
5. The cessation of the menstrual cycle in women is called _____.
6. _____ is often prescribed to women to reduce the negative effects of menopause.
7. Substances that some people believe cause sexual arousal are called _____.
8. A substance that can reduce sexual desire is called an _____.
9. The virus that causes AIDS is referred to as _____.
10. Avoiding sexual contact is called _____.
11. Having one sexual partner is referred to as being _____.
12. Insertion of the penis into the partner's mouth is called _____.

True-False Questions

1. _____ Human females are the only females capable of intense orgasmic response.
2. _____ Sexual equality between men and women has increased sexual dysfunctions for both because of the pressure to please the other partner.
3. _____ Many women who were early supporters of the women's movement now feel they have gained the right to say yes to their sexuality but have lost the right to say no to sexual advances.
4. _____ A study by Redbook found that for many men affection, tenderness, and cuddling were more important to their happiness than sex.
5. _____ Some women's sexual drive may become even stronger than the males in later years because of their multiorgasmic capability.
6. _____ In the early teens, females are more genitally oriented than males.
7. _____ Women have to learn how to reach orgasm but men do not.
8. _____ Women who experience multiple orgasms usually find their second and subsequent orgasmic episodes the most pleasurable.
9. _____ The size of the penis and the vagina greatly influence the experience of orgasm.
10. _____ Many sexologists consider masturbation to be an important and necessary part of sexual expression.
11. _____ The quality and quantity of the average couple's sex life are diminished by the daily chores of maintaining a family.
12. _____ Husbands tend to complain more than their wives about their children interfering with their sex lives.
13. _____ If men and women are sexually active in their early years, they tend to remain so in their later years.
14. _____ Alcohol increases the desire but decreases the performance.
15. _____ Men are more likely to acquire a sexually transmitted disease from women than women are from men.

Multiple-Choice Questions

1. When are females more sexually responsive?
    a. during ovulation
    b. just after the menstrual flow
    c. just before the menstrual flow
    d. it varies from woman to woman

2. Compared with other species, human sexuality is
    a. more a source of pleasure
    b. affected by learning and social factors
    c. less directly attached to reproduction
    d. all of the above

3. How have attitudes and behaviors in American society changed over the past thirty years?
   a. sexual expression has become freer, more diverse, and more open to public view
   b. the double standard is still strong
   c. homosexuality and bisexuality are more tolerated and accepted by the general public
   d. a better understanding of one's own sexuality is now an important goal, especially for men

4. What is the most important factor that has modified some of the changes brought about by freer sexual expression?
   a. recreational sex
   b. a change in values
   c. the epidemic return of sexually transmitted diseases
   d. none of the above

5. In a study by Psychology Today in 1994, what percentage of the respondents said they would not have sex with someone unless they were in love with them?
   a. 40
   b. 66
   c. 90
   d. 50

6. Puberty begins, on the average, _____ years earlier for females than males.
   a. 2
   b. 3
   c. 1
   d. 4

7. At what age(s) are males at the height of their sexual drive?
   a. 30
   b. 14
   c. 15 through the 20's
   d. 18

8. What does the research indicate about masturbation for men and women?
   a. women's and men's masturbation rates are lowest early in their lives
   b. women's masturbation rates increase slowly over the life span, while men's decrease
   c. men and women's masturbation rates are highest when they are young
   d. men and women's masturbation rates remain relatively stable over the life span

9. At what age(s) are females at the height of their sexual drive?
    a. 30 to 40
    b. 16 to 22
    c. 25 to 30
    d. 20 to 25

10. Sexually explicit material that has emotional and romantic overtones of sensuality and caring is referred to as
    a. pornography
    b. erotica
    c. X-rated
    d. promiscuity

11. Which is not one of the factors that changes fantasy content, as reported by Masters and Johnson?
    a. time
    b. personal experience
    c. gender
    d. one's culture

12. Masters and Johnson divided the sexual response cycle into four phases; they are, in order,
    a. plateau, excitement, orgasm, resolution
    b. excitement, orgasm, plateau, resolution
    c. excitement, plateau, resolution, orgasm
    d. excitement, plateau, orgasm, resolution

13. Which phase of the sexual response cycle is the most intense?
    a. excitement
    b. resolution
    c. orgasm
    d. plateau

14. In which phase of the sexual response cycle does tumescence and sex flush reach their peak?
    a. plateau
    b. excitement
    c. orgasm
    d. resolution

15. If orgasm does not occur, how long might the resolution phase last?
    a. 3 hours
    b. 12 hours or more
    c. 5 to 7 hours
    d. 1 to 3 hours

16. The refractory period may last only a few minutes or up to several hours depending on what factor?
    a. age
    b. health
    c. desire
    d. all of the above

17. Crook and Baur suggest that there may be three kinds of female orgasms; which is not one of the three?
    a. clitoral
    b. cervical
    c. uterine
    d. clitoral and uterine together

18. Wives tend to attribute their sexual problems to
    a. childbearing
    b. boredom
    c. fatigue
    d. stress

19. Happily married monogamous couples report greater sexual freedom because they are free from
    a. worry about pregnancy
    b. worry about STDs
    c. guilt associated with violating one's sexual standards
    d. all of the above

20. Which is not one of the criteria Masters and Johnson found for continuing sexual activity regardless of age?
    a. medication
    b. general health
    c. an interesting and interested sexual partner
    d. sexual organs must have regular use over the life span

21. Menopause generally occurs between the ages of
    a. 46 and 51
    b. 50 and 55
    c. 55 and 60
    d. 40 and 45

22. Estrogen replacement therapy is related to an increase in which type of cancer?
    a. cervical
    b. liver
    c. endometrium
    d. colon

23. What is the most widely used sexual stimulant in America?
    a. barbiturates
    b. alcohol
    c. amphetamines
    d. oysters

24. What is the most commonly reported communicable disease in the United Sates?
    a. herpes
    b. gonorrhea
    c. syphilis
    d. chlamydia

25. The disease that impairs the body's ability to fight infection is called
    a. gonorrhea
    b. hepatitis
    c. herpes
    d. AIDS

Critical Thinking and Decision Making
1. Identify the body changes that occur in the sexual response cycle.
2. After reviewing the authors findings about sexuality with respect to his classes, what are your biggest problems and complains about sexuality? Why?
3. Has the sexual revolution been beneficial for all ages, or just the young? Why?
4. We have prenuptial agreements, should we seriously consider a precoital contract? Why? Would you approach your potential partner with one?
5. Summarize the research on sexuality across the life span and in marriages.

Answers

Key Terms: 1   masturbation
              2   clitoris
              3   orgasm
              4   inhibited sexual desire
              5   menopause
              6   Estrogen Replacement therapy
              7   aphrodisiacs
              8   anaphrodisiacs
              9   human immunodeficiency virus
              10   abstinence
              11   monogamous
              12   fellatio

True/False: 1 T; 2 F; 3 T; 4 F; 5 T; 6 F; 7 T; 8 T; 9 F; 10 T; 11 T; 12 T; 13 T; 14 T; 15 F

Multiple Choice: 1 d; 2 d; 3 a; 4 c; 5 b; 6 a; 7 c; 8 b; 9 a; 10 b; 11 c; 12 d; 13 c; 14 a; 15 b; 16 d; 17 b; 18 c; 19 d; 20 a; 21 a; 22 c; 23 b; 24 b; 25 d

Chapter 11
Family Planning

Chapter Outline

- Family planning means controlling one's sexuality to avoid unwanted pregnancies and to create, when desired, an ideal family in which children can grow up in the healthiest possible manner.
- Years ago when the US was an agricultural nation, children were an economic asset because they helped to work the land. Today, the costs of raising children far outweigh their economic contributions. Therefore, the timing of children is often a major focus of family planning.
- The ideal family requires that:

  The children are wanted by both partners _____ .

  The partners are healthy enough physically & psychologically *to supply love & security to children*

  Family economic resources are adequate to nourish the children properly and keep them healthy.

  The family can supply the children with sufficient educational opportunity to acquire the skills necessary to survive and enjoy success within the culture.

Are We Ready For Children?

- Specific questions couples should address as they consider parenthood:

  How much time do we want for just each other and establishing a home?

  How much education do we want or need for the jobs and income we want?

  Are we ready to give a child the care, attention, and love she or he needs?

  Can we afford to provide our child with food, clothing, and education needed for at least 18 years?

  Can a child successfully fit into the lifestyle we feel is best for ourselves?

  What if we don't get the girl (boy) we want?

  What if the child is handicapped in some way?

Children Having Children

- A paradox of the last twenty years in the US: despite the availability of contraceptive devices, about 31 percent of all women having a child in 1992 were not married, up from 5 % in 1960.
- About 35 percent of children living with single parents live with a never-married parent.
- The percentage of women marrying before giving birth has dropped from 52% to 25 % from 1969 to 1993.
- Teen unwed pregnancies impose hardships:
    Teen mothers are many times more likely than older mothers to live below the poverty line.
    Only half of those giving birth before eighteen complete high school.
    Unwed mother earn about half as much money as older mothers.
- Children of unwed mothers have high rates of illness and mortality, often experience educational and emotional problems, are often victims of child abuse, and are prone to drop out of school and become teenage mothers themselves.
- The US leads nearly all developed nations in the incidence of pregnancy among girls aged 15 through 19.
- African American teenagers have the highest fertility rate of any teenage population in the world. One in four African American babies is born to a teen mother.
- The US spends $35 billion overall on income support for teenagers who are pregnant or have given birth.
- Researchers found that close parental supervision has the strongest influence in lowering the rate of childbearing in African American teenagers. For whites, high-quality relationships with parents was the strongest influence. For Hispanics, religiosity was the strongest.
- Newly active hormones coupled with the overwhelming sexual stimulation of the mass media and the sexual revolution mean teenagers will become pregnant unless parents and social institutions act to help them handle their sexuality.
- Fathers of teenagers' children tend to be in their twenties. Holding unwed fathers economically responsible for their children is only starting to be addressed.

Family Planning Decisions

- Women are having fewer children and are postponing both marriage and childbirth. Most women are now having their children at the ages of 25 and 34.
- The idea of birth control was mentioned in written records as far back as 1850 B.C.
- In 1873 Congress passed the Comstock Law which forbid the distribution of contraceptive information through the mail.
- Although many groups discourage the use of birth control, the vast majority of Americans practice birth control at some time.
- The ideal contraceptive does not exist. Such a contraceptive would be harmless, be reliable, be free from objectionable side effects, be inexpensive, be simple, be reversible in effect, be removed from the sexual act, and protect against venereal disease and AIDS.

- The condom is the third most used contraceptive after sterilization and the pill and is openly displayed on many store counters and vending machines. Latex condoms are nearly 100 percent effective against pregnancies and STDs. Condoms made of animal skin are permeable and do not protect against disease. Most pregnancies occur because of _Careless removal of the condom_ .
- Condoms for women are now available although relatively expensive.
- The diaphragm, which is obtained by prescription from a doctor, should be used with a spermicide, be inserted within two hours before intercourse, and be left in for six hours after intercourse. The main causes of pregnancies are _inaccurate fitting_ and _Incorrect insertion_ .
- The contraceptive sponge offered advantages over the diaphragm but was discontinued in 1994 because manufacturers could not meet new government safety rules.
- The intrauterine device (IUD) is inserted into the uterus by a doctor. It is second only to the pill in effectiveness. About 10 percent of women spontaneously expel them. About 2 to 3 percent of women develop pelvic inflammatory disease. In rare cases, the wall of the uterus may be punctured. Also, pelvic infections seem to be more common among IUD users.
- The pill is a combination of the hormones _estrogen_ and _progesterone_ and must be prescribed by a doctor. Taken daily, except for five days during menstruation, the pill stops ovulation. Its use declined as fear spread that it was linked to breast cancer, which fear seems unfounded by research. The most serious side effects include blood clots and possible increase in the risk of uterine cancer. Other side effects can be symptoms of early pregnancy, depression, nervousness, alteration of sex drive, dizziness, headaches, bleeding between periods, vaginal discharge, and yeast infections.
- The Norplant is a progestin-only implant under the skin of the inner upper arm that lasts for five years. It is relatively expensive at first, but averaged over five years is a cheap form of contraception.
- Three Month Contraception Injections, most commonly Depo-Prevara, are injections of progestin that last for three months.
- The Morning-After Pill contains hormones that prevent implantation of the egg if fertilization has taken place. Nausea and vomiting are frequent side effects. Also, menstrual irregularities, headaches, and dizziness are reported by users. Its full effects on the body many not be fully understood and should be the method of last resort.
- Rhythm requires the prediction of the four days during the menstrual cycle when conception can only occur and avoiding intercourse during those four days. Charting the menstrual cycle, charting the basal body temperature, and testing breath and saliva are means of determining the four day period. However, irregular cycles make rhythm unreliable, and about 15 percent of women are so irregular that rhythm can not be used at all.
- Vaginal spermicides are foams, creams, jellies, foaming tablets, and suppositories that contain sperm-killing agents which are placed in the vagina a short time before intercourse. Relatively harmless and easy to use, they are not very effective unless used with a diaphragm.
- Withdrawal (coitus interruptus) is withdrawal of the male just before ejaculation. It has a high failure rate.

- Sterilization is the most effective and permanent means of birth control. Vasectomies involve cutting and tying the vasa deferentia of the male. Tubal ligation involves the cutting and tying of the fallopian tubes of the female. Laparoscopy involves the same procedure but radio waves, using a small tube, severe the tubes, and therefore is a much simpler and quicker procedure. A hysterectomy is the surgical removal of the uterus and is used for other problems of the uterus, not just for birth control. Reversals of vasectomies and tubal ligations are possible in the majority of cases.

Abortion

- After a number of states liberalized abortion laws, the US Supreme Court in *Roe vs. Wade and Doe vs. Bolton* made abortion on request a possibility in 1973 for the entire country.
- The Court ruled that states _that the fetus is not a person_ during the first trimester, may lay down medical guidelines to protect the mother's health during the second trimester, and can ban abortions during the third trimester.
- The Court essentially ruled that the fetus is not a citizen and is therefore not protected by the Constitution.
- Abortion is one of the most emotional issues the nation faces with the country fairly evenly divided on the question of allowing abortions. The arguments revolve around: when does life begin?
- In 1992, the US Supreme Court again upheld *Roe vs. Wade* and further restricted that:
    Women seeking abortions must be told about fetal development and alternatives to ending pregnancies.
    Women must wait _24_ hours after receiving that information before proceeding with an abortion.
    Doctors are required to keep detailed records, subject to public disclosure, on each abortion performed.
    Unmarried girls under 18 and not supporting themselves are required to get consent of one of their parents or the permission of a state judge who has ruled the girl is mature enough to make the decision on her own.
- Another aspect of the abortion debate concerns the right of the father to participate in the abortion decision. Current laws exclude him from the decision.
- Improving medical technology also influences the abortion debate. Now, technology allows the fetus to survive outside the womb as early as 24 weeks, and some doctors predict it will soon be 20 weeks.
- Methods of abortion include:
    Dilatation and curettage (D and C) in which the contents of the uterus are scraped out.
    Vacuum aspiration in which vacuum is used to remove the contents of the uterus.
    RU-486 (not available in the US) in which a pill or suppository induces expulsion of the embryo.
    Saline abortion, used after the fourteenth to sixteenth week, in which the fetus is killed with an injection of saline and the body then rejects the dead fetus.
- Abortion is <u>not</u> recommended as a means of birth control.

Infertility
- About _one_ in twelve couples have problems conceiving.
- _Infertile_ means the man is not producing viable sperm or the woman is not producing viable eggs.
- Age has a moderate effect on fertility and does not begin in women until the late thirties. Women are born with their entire supply of eggs and no more are produced. With time, the eggs age, and the number of viable eggs are reduced.
- _Young_ : partners have the capacity to reproduce.
- Males and females each account for about 40 percent of fertility problems. In the remaining 20 percent, both members account for the problem.
- Infertility in males may involve impotence, low sperm count, testes that have not descended into the scrotum, and STDs.
- Infertility in females may involve not releasing an egg, a blocked tract from the vagina though the uterus to the Fallopian tubes, vaginal infections, ovarian abnormalities, and STDs.
- Infertility may be treated by artificial insemination, fertility drugs, artificial fertilization and embryo transfer, the use of surrogate mothers, and sex therapy.

Summary
- Family planning is an important part of marriage.
- The pill, IUD, condom, sterilization, and diaphragm are all popular and effective methods of birth control.
- Sterilization as a form of birth control has become increasingly popular.
- Abortion laws have been revised, making abortion on demand a reality.
- Family planning also helps couples have children when fertility problems exist.

Key Terms
1. Any devise or drug used to prevent pregnancy is called a _contraceptive_.
2. A sheath designed to cover the penis during sexual intercourse is called a _condom_.
3. The _diaphragm_ is a dome-shape cup of thin latex measured to fit the vagina.
4. The _cervical cap_ is a small dome-shaped cup of thin latex used to fit over the cervix.
5. A soft , round polyurethane sponge permeated with spermicide is called a _contraceptive sponge_
6. A small object inserted into a woman's uterus to prevent conception is called an _intrauterine device_.
7. An _ectopic pregnancy_ is the implantation of the fertilized egg in one of the fallopian tubes.
8. A six capsule progestin-only implant that provides up to 5 years of contraceptive protection is called _norplant_.
9. An injection of progestin which provides protection for three months is called _3 mon. contraceptive injection_
10. Pills that are taken after intercourse to prevent implantation of the fertilized egg are called _morning after pill_.

11. The _rhythm_ method of contraception that is based on abstinence during the time of ovulation.
12. The _basal body temperature_ method of contraception is based on the lowest body temperature of a person.
13. Foams, creams, jellies, tablets, and suppositories are examples of _spermicides_.
14. The _withdrawal_ method is where the male removes the penis before ejaculation.
15. The most effective and permanent means of birth control is _sterilization_.
16. Termination of a pregnancy before the fetus is capable of surviving on its own is called _abortion_.
17. The inability to gain or maintain an erection is called _impotence_.
18. Injecting sperm from a husband or donor into a woman's vagina is called _artificial insemination_.
19. _Fertility drugs_ are used to help overstimulate the ovaries to produce multiple eggs.
20. Transferring fertilized eggs to a woman's uterus is called _in vitro fertilization_ or _embryo transfer_.
21. Intervention used to help couples with their sexual problems and the ability to conceive is called _sex therapy_.

True-False Questions

1. __T__ The decision to have children is one of the most important family decisions, yet it is often made haphazardly or not made at all.
2. __T__ Only half of the females who give birth before eighteen complete high school.
3. __T__ The main causes of pregnancy when using a diaphragm are inaccurate fitting and incorrect insertion.
4. __F__ After a vasectomy men's hormone production decreases, causing a slight decrease in sex drive.
5. __T__ The decision to have an abortion should be reached as quickly as possible since the longer one waits, the greater the risks of complications.
6. __T__ Men and women, each, account for about 40 percent of the infertility problems; 20 percent of the time, both account for infertility problems.
7. __T__ The percentage of children conceived out of wedlock has not risen substantially from 1960 to now, but the percentage of women marrying before the birth has dropped significantly.
8. __F__ Tubal ligations are cheaper and easier to perform than vasectomies.
9. __F__ No state can interfere in any way with a woman's right to have an abortion up to 25 weeks; after that, states can lay down medical guidelines to protect the woman's health.
10. __F__ The abortion ratio for black women is 4 times that of white women.
11. __T__ When the cause of infertility rests with the husband, artificial insemination is often used.

Multiple-Choice Questions

1. Which is not one of the reasons why women have high rates of unwanted pregnancies when we have more birth control methods?
    a. they are unrealistically romantic about sex
    b. they hesitate to inconvenience their partner
    c. they are proud of their sexuality
    d. they believe it can't happen to them

2. Which of the following is not one of the possible effects of teenage pregnancy?
    a. abuse of the child
    b. low rates of infant mortality
    c. the mother drops out of school
    d. emotional problems for the mother

3. According to a study done by the Guttmacher Institute of thirty-seven countries, which country has the highest incidence of teenage pregnancy?
    a. United States
    b. Sweden
    c. France
    d. Britain

4. Studies indicate that females wait approximately how long after initiating sexual intercourse before they seek contraception?
    a. 6 months
    b. 18 months
    c. 8 months
    d. 12 months

5. According to the Guttmacher Institute, who has the highest fertility rate of any teenage population in the entire world?
    a. Asians
    b. Caucasians
    c. African Americans
    d. Native American Indian

6. What percent of pregnant teens become pregnant again within one year?
    a. 50 %
    b. 25 %
    c. 15 %
    d. 30 %

7. According to the Rand Corporation study that looked at adolescent pregnancy, what was the strongest predictor among black teens for lowering the rate of single childbearing?
   a. close parental supervision
   b. high quality relationship with parents
   c. being over 16
   d. religious beliefs

8. According to the Rand Corporation study that looked at adolescent pregnancy, what was the strongest predictor among whites for lowering the rate of single childbearing?
   a. religious beliefs
   b. high quality relationship with parents
   c. close parental supervision
   d. education about birth control

9. The majority of women are now having their children between the ages of
   a. 20 and 30
   b. 18 and 25
   c. 30 and 40
   d. 25 and 34

10. An ideal birth control method should:
   a. be highly effective in preventing pregnancy
   b. be inexpensive
   c. protect againsts STDs
   d. all of the above

11. In today's society, the greatest advantage of using the condom is
   a. it's effectiveness
   b. ease of use
   c. protection against AIDS and sexually transmitted diseases
   d. minimal side effects

12. What is the third most popular contraceptive method?
   a. pill
   b. norplant
   c. condom
   d. IUD

13. A new device that is made of a soft, loose-fitting polyurethane sheath and two diaphragm-like, flexible rings is called a
    a. female condom
    b. diaphragm
    c. sponge
    d. cervical cap

14. Which contraceptive should be checked every two years, and after childbirth, an abortion, or after a weight gain or loss of ten or more pounds?
    a. cervical cap
    b. IUD
    c. norplant
    d. diaphragm

15. Which contraceptive is associated with pelvic inflammatory disease?
    a. pill
    b. norplant
    c. IUD
    d. depo-provera

16. The pill offers protection against all but one of the following
    a. breast cysts
    b. uterine cancer
    c. ovarian cancer
    d. pelvic inflammatory disease

17. Which of the following is the most effect type of spermicide?
    a. creams
    b. jellies
    c. foams
    d. suppositories

18. Which is believed to be the oldest form of birth control?
    a. sterilization
    b. coitus interruptus
    c. condom
    d. diaphragm

19. Which is the most popular form of birth control?
    a. sterilization
    b. pill
    c. norplant
    d. condom

20. Studies indicate what percent of vasectomies are reversible?
    a. 20 to 30 %
    b. 40 to 50 %
    c. 85 to 100 %
    d. 50 to 90 %

21. For white women the greatest number of abortions occur at _____ years of age; for African-Americans it is _____ years of age?
    a. 23 and 21
    b. 18 and 21
    c. 16 and 18
    d. 17 and 18

22. In June of 1992, the Supreme Court upheld Roe vs. Wade, but placed restrictions on abortions. Which is not one of the restrictions?
    a. doctors detailed records are not open to public disclosure
    b. unmarried girls under 18 and not supporting themselves are required to obtain parental consent or a judge must render her mature enough to make the decision
    c. women must be told about fetal development and alternatives
    d. women must wait 24 hours after receiving information to obtain the abortion

23. Ninety-six percent of all abortions are done by this method; it is
    a. dilation and curettage
    b. saline abortion
    c. RU-486
    d. vacuum aspiration

24. The type of abortion where amniotic fluid is removed and a salt solution is put in the amniotic sac to induce delivery is called
    a. D and C
    b. saline abortion
    c. vacuum aspiration
    d. RU-486

25. Couples are considered infertile if they have unprotected intercourse for _____ and do not conceive.
    a. 2 years
    b. 6 months
    c. 1 year
    d. 8 months

Critical Thinking and Decision Making

1. Unmarried females have three options when they become pregnant, abort, keep the child, or give it up for adoption. If you became an unwed mother, which option would you choose and why?
2. Compare and contrast the types of birth control with respect to side effects. Which is the least harmful to the body, but offers the most protection?
3. If you and your spouse were infertile, which childbearing alternative would you use? Why?
4. Discuss the pros and cons of abortion?
5. Discuss the moral and ethical issues of the infertility treatments? Are we really dealing with something that should be left alone?

Answers
Key Terms: 1   contraceptive
2   condom
3   diaphragm
4   cervical cap
5   contraceptive sponge
6   Intrauterine device
7   ectopic pregnancy
8   norplant
9   three month contraceptive injection
10   morning after pill
11   rhythm
12   basal body temperature
13   spermicides
14   withdrawal
15   sterilization
16   abortion
17   impotence
18   artificial insemination
19   fertility drugs
20   invitro fertilization or embryo transfer
21   sex therapy

True/False: 1 T; 2 T; 3 T; 4 F; 5 T; 6 T; 7 T; 8 F; 9 F; 10 F; 11 T

Multiple Choice: 1 c; 2 b; 3 a; 4 d; 5 c; 6 c; 7 a; 8 b; 9 d; 10 d; 11 c; 12 c; 13 a; 14 d; 15 c; 16 b; 17 c; 18 b; 19 a; 20 d; 21 b; 22 a; 23 d; 24 b; 25 c

Chapter 12
Pregnancy and Birth

Chapter Outline

- Although women of the 1950s felt social pressure to marry and have children, the pressure slowly dissipated, and today childlessness is much more accepted.

Conception

- About 200 to 400 million sperm are produced in an average ejaculation. Sperm swim from the vagina to the Fallopian tube that contains the egg where one of them fertilizes the egg. Once fertilized, the egg begins to move down the Fallopian tube to the uterus.
- Sperm remain viable within the female reproductive tract about 48 hours; the egg remains viable for about 24 hours.
- The female egg always carries an X chromosome; the sperm may carry an X or Y chromosome. If the egg is fertilized by an X sperm, the child will be female; if it is fertilized by a Y sperm, it will be male.
- About _140_ males are conceived for every_100_females. However, only _106_ males are born for every 100 females.
- Normally a female conceives one child at a time. Mortality rates are much higher for multiple births.
- _Fraternal_ twins are developed from two separate eggs that are fertilized simultaneously.
- _Identical_ twins are developed when a single fertilized egg subdivides.

Pregnancy

- Some common early signs of pregnancy are a missed menstrual period, morning sickness, changes in shape and coloration of the breasts, increased need to urinate, feelings of fatigue and sleepiness, increased vaginal secretions, and increased retention of body fluids.

- Pregnancy tests are considered _95_ to _98_ percent reliable. Performed either by doctors or through inexpensive home kits, they test for agglutination, the clumping together of human chorionic gonadotrophin. (HCG).
- False pregnancy occurs when early physical signs of pregnancy are present but the woman is not really pregnant.
- The average duration of pregnancy is _266_ days. / 38 weeks
- The developing baby is called an _embryo_ for the first two months; after that it is called a _fetus_ .
- _Congenital_ defects are birth defects caused by negative influences from outside.
- _Genetic_ defects are birth defects inherited through genes.
- The fetus receives nourishment from the mother's blood through the umbilical cord and placenta, although there is no direct intermingling of blood.
- Many drugs taken by the mother can cause birth defects. If addictive drugs are used, the child will be born addicted and suffer withdrawal symptoms.
- Other causes of damage to the fetus include infectious diseases, smoking, alcohol, radiation, and Rh blood diseases.
- Regular prenatal visits with a physician are important to assure good health of the child. Prenatal care may involve:

  Diet: assuring the mother eats a well-balanced diet.

  Amniocentesis: testing for genetic defects.

  Utrasound: testing to learn about the position, size, and state of development of the fetus.

  Fetoscopy: direct examination of the fetus by inserting a small tube in the amniotic sac.
- Intercourse normally poses no real threat but should be avoided during the last three weeks of pregnancy.

Birth
- After nine months of pregnancy, the woman has probably gained twenty to twenty-five pounds. The baby is usually 7 to 8 pounds of the weight.
- Two reasons for not gaining excessive weight are _excessive weight can strain the circ._ and the difficulty to lose the extra weight. However, dieting during pregnancy carries the risk of robbing the fetus of good nutrition.
- Pregnancies range from 240 to 300 days; there is only a 50 percent chance that birth will occur within one week of the expected birth date.
- Labor occurs in three stages:

  1. Lasting from 8 to 20 hours, the cervix dilates enough for the baby to pass, the sac of amniotic fluid breaks, and contractions begin.

  2. Lasting from 15 minutes to an hour or so, called the transition, the child is pushed down through the vagina.

  3. Lasting from 5 to 20 minutes, the afterbirth, or detached placenta, is delivered.

- If the baby is too large to pass through the mother's pelvis or labor is very long and hard, the baby may be removed by cesarean section in which an incision is made through the abdominal and uterine walls, and the baby is removed.
- The majority of pain arises from pressure of the baby's head against the cervix, the opening of the birth canal.
- Episiotomy involves making a small incision in the skin between the vaginal and anal openings to avoid tearing of the skin during birth.
- Natural childbirth means the mother has a good understanding of birth procedures, not simply childbirth without anesthesia. General anesthesia has become much less popular because it slows labor and depresses the child's activity. More and more physicians are allowing the woman to decide whether she wants an anesthetic and if so, what type.
- More and more hospitals are allowing the mother to keep her baby with her rather than placing it in a nursery. This is called Rooming - in .
- Some hospitals have created alternative birth centers, a homelike setting in which birth occurs and relatives and friends are allowed to visit during much of the birthing process.
- Less than one percent of all births occur in a private home (called National U.S. Center for Health Statistics). Midwives are used in home delivery in many modern countries.
- The natural childbirth philosophy has emphasized breast feeding because it is more natural; it brings the mother and child into close, physical contact which encourages bonding; close contact develops security and basic trust in the infant; colostrum which is high in antibodies is present in the mother's milk for a few days after birth; breastfeeding speeds the uterus's return to normal; and nursing mothers experience warm, loving feelings.
- The postpartum period is the first few weeks and months after childbirth. About 60 percent of women report mild emotional depression and 10 percent report severe depression. For most women, this depression passes within a few days after childbirth.

Summary
- Pregnancy and childbirth are an integral part of most marriages.
- Both the egg and sperm cells are among the smallest in the body, yet they contain all the genetic material necessary to create the adult human being.
- Pregnancy takes several weeks before it is recognizable, though some pregnancy tests can determine pregnancy within seven to ten days of conception.
- The average pregnancy is 266 days, or 36 weeks.
- The birth process is generally divided into three stages.
- In recent years more and more emphasis has been placed on having the mother and father participate as much as they can in the birth of the child.
- Philosophically, those encouraging natural childbirth believe that for a couple to share the miracle of creating life can be an emotional high point.

Key Terms

1. The number of children born each year is called the _birthrate_.
2. The moment of fertilization of the egg by the sperm is called _conception_.
3. The hollow organ in females in which the fetus develops is called the _uterus_.
4. Twins who develop from two separate eggs are called _fraternal_.
5. Twins who develop from one egg that divides after fertilization are called _identical_.
6. When physical signs of pregnancy appear but a woman is not pregnant it is called _pseudocyesis / false pregnancy_.
7. The first two months after conception the organism is called an _embryo_.
8. From the second month to the ninth month of prenatal development, the organism is called a _fetus_.
9. Negative elements from the outside environment sometimes cause birth defects, these defects are referred to as _congenital defects_.
10. Birth defects caused by the genes are called ~~umbilical cord, placenta~~ _genetic defects_.
11. Nourishment from the mother is passed to the fetus through the ~~Rh factor~~ and the ~~amniocentesis~~ _Rh factor_. _umbilical cord, placenta_
12. A chemical, named for the rhesus monkey, that lies on the surface of the red blood cells is called the ~~ultrasound~~ _Rh factor_.
13. The procedure of removing amniotic fluid from the amniotic sac to determine any birth defects is called ~~fetoscopy~~ _aminocentesis_.
14. The procedure of using sound waves to view the developing fetus for structural problems is called an ~~fetus~~ _ultrasound_.
15. Examining the fetus through a small viewing tube inserted into the mother's uterus is called a _fetoscopy_.
16. Preparation for delivering a child where the uterus contracts and the cervix dilates is called _labor_.
17. The fluid that surrounds the fetus in the uterus is called the _amniotic fluid_.
18. _transition_ occurs when the fetus moves from the uterus into the vagina.
19. A small incision made between the vaginal opening and the anal opening is called an _episiotomy_.
20. A birth process where women have been educated and are taught breathing and relaxation techniques is known as _natural child birth_.
21. The concept of allowing the child to remain in the same room with the mother after delivery is known as _rooming-in_.
22. A homelike setting for childbirth that is created by hospitals is called _alternative birth centers_.
23. Delivering a child at home is called a _home birth_.
24. Professionals who deliver babies at home are called _midwives_.
25. The first milk secreted by the breast feeding mother is called _colostrum_.

True-False Questions

1. ____T____ A male must ejaculate millions of sperm because the task of reaching the egg is so arduous that only a few thousand ever reach the fallopian tube and the egg.
2. ____T____ Conception can only occur during approximately three days of each twenty-eight day cycle.
3. ____F____ Females determine the gender of the child by supplying either an X or Y chromosome.
4. ____F____ More females are conceived and born than males.
5. ____F____ Most twins are identical.
6. ____T____ The menstrual cycle is easily altered by one's emotions.
7. ____F____ First born children are at greatest risk for complications from the Rh factor.
8. ____T____ Because the uterine contractions of orgasm are similar to labor contractions, intercourse should be avoided during the last three weeks of pregnancy.
9. ____T____ Intercourse poses no real threat to most pregnancies because contractions from orgasms can strengthen the uterine muscles.
10. ____T____ Fetal weight above nine pounds complicates labor and delivery and increases the risk of postpartum hemorrhage.
11. ____F____ Natural childbirth is more traumatic to the mother's body than cesarean section births.

Multiple-Choice Questions

1. Fertilization must occur within _____ hours of ovulation or the egg will die and be expelled.
   a. 36
   b. 12
   c. 24
   d. 48

2. Sperm remain viable within the female reproductive tract for about
   a. 36 hours
   b. 48 hours
   c. 24 hours
   d. 12 hours

3. The inner cells that surround the fertilized egg separate into three layers. The middle layer becomes the
   a. muscles, bone, blood, kidneys, and sex glands
   b. skin, hair, and nervous tissue
   c. endoderm
   d. ectoderm

4. Which of the following is not one of the signs of pregnancy?
    a. missed menstrual period
    b. increased vaginal secretions
    c. changes in shape and coloration of breasts
    d. increased acne

5. Pregnancy tests are looking for the presence of what substance in a women's urine to verify pregnancy?
    a. estrogen
    b. human chorionic gonadotropin
    c. pseudocyesis
    d. testosterone

6. The best known infectious disease contracted by the mother which may harm the fetus is
    a. herpes
    b. chicken pox
    c. German measles
    d. syphilis

7. What is one of the major predictors of infant death?
    a. low birth weight
    b. fetal alcohol syndrome
    c. Rh blood disease
    d. none of the above

8. In a health department study, which group of women had the highest rates of smoking while pregnant?
    a. African Americans
    b. Hispanics
    c. Asians
    d. American Indians

9. The US Public Health Service suggests _____ may be the leading cause of birth defects in the US.
    a. Rh factor
    b. smoking
    c. German measles
    d. alcohol

10. Which of the following prenatal tests allows the doctor to directly view the fetus through an endoscope?
    a. amniocentesis
    b. fetoscopy
    c. ultrasound
    d. all of the above

11. An ultrasound allows a doctor to learn about all of the following but one, it is
    a. internal problems
    b. position of fetus
    c. size of fetus
    d. structural problems

12. Guidelines issued by the National Academy of Sciences advises an optimum weight gain of _____ for women.
    a. 20-25 pounds
    b. 30-40 pounds
    c. 25-35 pounds
    d. 35-40 pounds

13. Which stage of labor and delivery lasts the longest?
    a. first stage
    b. second stage
    c. transition
    d. third stage

14. The _____ stage of labor and delivery is when the child is born.
    a. first
    b. second
    c. transition
    d. third

15. The incidence of infection associated with a cesarean delivery is about _____ times higher than with vaginal deliveries.
    a. 1 to 3
    b. 3 to 5
    c. 10 to 15
    d. 5 to 10

16. The majority of pain occurs during which stage of labor and delivery?
     a. first
     b. second
     c. transition
     c. third

17. Women can reduce the pain of labor by doing all but one of the following.
     a. breathing shallowly
     b. lying on her back
     c. lying in a fetal position
     d. relaxing at the onset of a contraction

18. Natural childbirth is defined as
     a. no medication during labor and delivery
     b. childbirth with very little pain
     c. education and breathing and relaxation techniques
     d. none of the above

19. The major reason psychologists advocate breast feeding is
     a. it encourages bonding between mother and child
     b. it is more natural
     c. the child receives the colostrum
     d. the uterus returns to its normal size faster

20. About _____ percent of all women report a mild degree of emotional depression following childbirth.
     a. 10
     b. 60
     c. 50
     d. 80

21. Women who attend childbirth classes report experiencing _____ during labor and delivery
     than women who don't attend the classes.
     a. more pain
     b. less pain
     c. the same amount of pain
     d. no research has been conducted

22. Which of the following is not one of the three layers of the fertilized egg?
    a. endoderm
    b. ectoderm
    c. mesoderm
    d. plasoderm

23. Poor diets in pregnant women can cause which of the following problems in the fetus?
    a. stunted growth
    b. rickets
    c. mental retardation
    d. all of the above

24. The average labor for first born children is _____, while the average for subsequent children is _____.
    a. 8 to 20; 3 to 8
    b. 6 to 8; 4 to 6
    c. 12 to 24; 8 to 10
    d. 15 to 20; 10 to 12

25. Which of the following is not one of the basic principles underlying natural childbirth?
    a. education reduces fear and less fear means less tension and pain
    b. breathing and relaxation techniques alleviate some of the pain
    c. women should never be given medication
    d. mothers and fathers should be active participants in childbirth

Critical Thinking and Decision Making
1. Do you agree with the author in that the unborn child is an aware, reacting being? Why?
2. Compare and contrast the prenatal tests for benefits and risks.
3. If you were going to have a prenatal test, which one would you choose and why?
4. What are the advantages and disadvantages of the types of environments a child can be born into? Which environment would you choose and why?
5. What are the advantages and disadvantages of breast feeding versus bottle feeding?

Answers

Key Terms:

	1	birthrate
	2	conception
	3	uterus
	4	fraternal
	5	identical
	6	pseudocyesis or false pregnancy
	7	embryo
	8	fetus
	9	congenital defects
	10	genetic defects
	11	umbilical cord; placenta
	12	Rh factor
	13	amniocentesis
	14	ultrasound
	15	fetoscopy
	16	labor
	17	amniotic fluid
	18	transition
	19	episiotomy
	20	natural childbirth
	21	rooming-in
	22	alternative birth centers
	23	home birth
	24	midwives
	25	colostrum

True/False: 1 T; 2 T; 3 F; 4 F; 5 F; 6 T; 7 F; 8 T; 9 T; 10 T; 11 F

Multiple Choice: 1 c; 2 b; 3 a; 4 d; 5 b; 6 c; 7 a; 8 d; 9 d; 10 b; 11 a; 12 c; 13 a; 14 b; 15 d; 16 c; 17 b; 18 c; 19 a; 20 b; 21 b; 22 d; 23 d; 24 a; 25 c

Chapter 13
The Challenge of Parenthood

Chapter Outline

- In the past, many popular assumptions supported the having of children:
    Marriage means children.
    Having children is the essence of a women's self-realization.
    Reproduction is a woman's biological destiny.
    All families have a duty to have children to replenish society.
    Children prove the manliness of the father.
    Children prove the competence and womanliness of the mother.
    Humans should be fruitful and multiply.
    Having children is humanity's way to immortality.
    Children are an economic asset.
- The assumptions of the past have become the liability of today because uncontrolled reproduction now means the ultimate demise of the species.

Children by Choice

- Wrong reasons for having children include _____ , pleasing parents or friends, _____ , escaping from the outside working world, relieving loneliness, wanting to do a better job than your parents did, and proving that you are a real man or woman.
- While remaining childless has become more acceptable by our society, women are feeling the new pressure of advancing age and having children before it is too late.
- Childlessness has numerous advantages, the most important of which is freedom.

What Effects Do Children Have On A Marriage?
- Parenthood is demanding and lasts until the end of your life.
- Transition to parenthood involves a number of costs to parents:

  _____ .

  Unforeseen strains are placed on the husband-wife relationship.
  The personal elements of the marital relationship tend to become less satisfying.
  Children place new limits on social lives.
- About _____ of parents report that children were their main satisfaction in life.
- Except for two-career families that can afford to place child care almost entirely in the hands of others, the parents' relationship moves in the traditional direction, i.e. the mother turns to parenting and household roles while the father turns toward the work world.
- Studies have shown that even when a mother returns to work, her employment has a negligible impact on the husband's housework and child-care responsibilities.
- The historical characterization of the harsh, austere, disciplinarian father is being replaced by the more humanistic, affectionate, caring father.
- In _____ percent of the cases, children go with their mother when families break up. Fathering is drastically reduced, and fathers' contact with children declines rapidly.
- Some researchers believe that America's most urgent social problem is lack of fathering.

Stimulation and Development
- Stimulation is necessary for the development of basic behavioral capacities. Key dimension of mothering offer stimulation: physical contact, attentiveness, verbal stimulation, material stimulation, responsive care, and some restrictiveness.
- The preschool years are important to the cognitive development of the child.
- Some stress in a child's life is beneficial to development of stress tolerance.
- Parents are sources of stimulation to children by speaking to and playing with infants. They are mediators or filters of stimulation by directing the infant's attention to objects and events and by restricting the toddler from engaging in dangerous activities.

Parental Effectiveness
- There is little agreement about the best way to rear children. Parental growth and development go hand in hand with child growth and development.
- Research indicates that cultural groups are more similar than they are different in rearing children, although ethnic parents tend to be stricter.
- Studies show that the _____ parenting style relates most closely to producing competent children. This style emphasized the development of autonomy and independence in children with reasonable parental limits.
- Neglect and lack of parenting is a far bigger problem than overprotection since children will not have enough contact to copy proper behavior.

- Our economic system, schools, religious organizations, mass media, and many other institutions and groups influence children's development.
- By age seventeen, most children have spent more time watching television than going to school.
- The _____ of 1992 regulated advertising in children's programs, required specific TV programs to meet the needs of children, and gave examples of acceptable children's programs.
- Anderson and Collins found that:

  _____ .

  _____ .

  Television generally displaces movies, radio, comic books and sports rather than general reading.

  Homework done while watching television is of no lower quality than homework done in silence.

  Television does not reduce children's attention span but may actually increase their ability to focus attention.

  Television may reduce reading achievement but, if so, occurs during early elementary school years and is probably temporary.

- The potential for good in television is as large as its potential for harm. Parents may need to set rules for their children's television viewing: the amount of time for viewing, the actual time of day or evening for viewing, the types of programs for viewing, the amount of adult attention during and after viewing, and whether television will be used as a reward to influence other behavior.
- Among three and four year olds, researchers found a strong correlation between physical aggression and frequent viewing of all but educational children's programs. Prosocial behavior and the use of mature language was related to viewing educational children's programs.
- Besides leading to aggressive behavior, television viewing may also lead to problems in holding children's attention when complex issues require deep study and in depriving children of important social interactions.
- Persons who fail to internalize social rules and mores are called _____ . As adults, they show a conspicuous lack of parenting.
- Risk behavior that leads to antisocial personality disorders are:

  Parent withdraws and assumes negative psychological and physical posture regarding the baby at birth.

  Minimal touching, stroking, or talking to or about the baby unless in a negative manner.

  Parent has emotionless or flat effect or is often depressed and angry.

  Parent overstimulates the child by too much talking or play in inappropriate or hostile ways.

  Parent doesn't establish eye contact except when angry and rarely smiles or does so inappropriately such as when the child is in pain.

  _____ .

  _____ .

  Mother is unhappy, frustrated, and angry at being a mother and primary caretaker.

Childrearing, Discipline, and Control
- Most parents overwhelmingly use negative techniques such as scolding, spanking, and threatening to control their children. Unfortunately, negative techniques tend to have negative side effects because they serve as model behavior.
- Childrearing should be a rational, thoughtful, directive process rather than an irrational, reactive process. Milder methods of control that could be effective are preferred to stronger methods.

The Growing Child in the Family
- Change and growth in the child mean parental and family change:
    Infancy: The Oral-Sensory Stage: Trust Versus Mistrust (First Year)
        Children are completely dependent on parents and other.
    Toddler: The Muscular-Anal Stage: Autonomy Versus Shame and Doubt (2 to 3 years old)
        First steps, first words and curiosity make this a period of quick change.
    Early Childhood: The Locomoter-Genital Stage: Initiative Versus Guilt (4 to 5 years old)
        Children become increasingly capable of self-initiated activities.
    School Age: The Latency Stage: Industry Versus Inferiority (6 to 11 years old)
        Children become interesting, more individual, and increasingly independent.
    The Puberty: Adolescence Stage: Identity Versus Role Diffusion (12 to 18 years old)
        Peer influence becomes stronger than parental influence.
    The Young Adulthood Stage: Intimacy Versus Isolation
        Parents often continue to support their children after schooling.
- The problems of puberty and adolescence fall into four main categories:
    _____ .
    _____ .
    Forming good peer group relations.
    Developing goals and a philosophy of life.

Broader Parenting
- Some critics argue that the nuclear family pattern of parents and children always alone together creates problems in children rather than preventing them. Trading care of children with other families, setting up volunteer community nursery schools, establishing business-supplied-day-care, and expanding the nuclear family to include relatives are broader parenting alternatives.

Parents Without Pregnancy: Adoption
- _____ percent of babies placed for adoption are born of never-married mothers. More babies are probably available today for adoption than in the early 1970s.
- Adoption costs range from $5,000 to $20,000.
- A unique parenting problem faced by adoptive parents is that of deciding whether and when to tell the child that he/she is adopted. Experts believe the best course is to inform the child from the beginning.

- Many adoptive children feel the need to know something about their natural parents.
- Cooperative adoption involves the biological parents and adoptive parents mutually working out the adoption.

The Single-Parent Family

- The single-parent family is the fastest growing type in the US. The majority are women and their children. Larger amounts of welfare aid goes to single-parent families headed by women which indicates the financial difficulties they face.
- Social and emotional isolation are two major problems facing a single parent.

Summary

- Parenthood remains one of the major functions of marriage.
- Parenthood is a difficult and ever-changing job that demands intelligence, flexibility, emotional warmth, stability, and a good portion of courage.
- Children will affect their parents in many ways.
- Erik Erikson identifies eight psychosocial developmental stages that describe the human life cycle from infancy through old age.
- Broader parenting would help parents do a better job.
- Adoption is another avenue to parenthood.
- The single-parent family, although usually transitory, is more common today than ever before.

Key Terms

1. Children who spend part of their day without adult supervision are called _____.
2. The period in which children experience biological changes and mature sexually is called

   _____.
3. The time period in which children deal with social and cultural influences that assist them in becoming adults is called _____.

True-False Questions

1. _____ By reducing infant mortality, we have removed the necessity for most American families to have large numbers of children.
2. _____ A couple's conscious or unconscious reasons for having children strongly affects the way children are treated and reared.
3. _____ Women are postponing marriage and childbirth and are having fewer children.
4. _____ Remaining childless after marriage is more accepted today, although childless couples still feel they are viewed negatively by others.
5. _____ The key factor in whether children experience negative effects from mother absence and child care is the quality of the care.

6. _____ Marital satisfaction increases when children enter the home.
7. _____ Most parents express overall satisfaction with children and the parenting role.
8. _____ Parents become less traditional in their gender role behaviors when children enter the home.
9. _____ Fathers tend to be more involved with their daughters than with their sons.
10. _____ Of all the types of abuse and neglect, physical abuse is the greatest problem.
11. _____ Most parents overwhelmingly use positive techniques to control their children.
12. _____ During the adolescent stage, peer influence becomes stronger than parental influence.
13. _____ Many single parent families are a transitional family form.
14. _____ Adolescents with the fewest economic and social resources are most likely to offer their child for adoption.

Multiple-Choice Questions

1. Which of the following is not one of the wrong reasons to have a child?
   a. to save or strengthen a marriage
   b. you think children are fun
   c. to do a better job then your parents did
   d. to please parents

2. Why do unwed teenage mothers keep their children?
   a. to have something of their own
   b. because they love children
   c. because they feel they are ready to be parents
   d. to prove to the world they are fertile

3. The most important advantage of being a childless couple is
   a. career opportunities
   b. monetarily less encumbered
   c. time for themselves
   d. increased freedom

4. What does the research indicate about childless and parental couples in terms of cohesion?
   a. parental couples have higher levels of cohesion
   b. their is no difference between the two couples on cohesion
   c. childless couples have higher levels of cohesion
   d. the research is inconclusive

5. The parent/child relationship is best described as
    a. parents socialize children
    b. parents socialize children and children socialize parents
    c. children socialize parents
    d. children only complicate marriages

6. The transition to parenthood involves many costs to the parents, one of which is
    a. less time for socializing
    b. less discretionary income
    c. romance and sex become less satisfying
    d. all of the above

7. Parents identify which of the following as a benefit of having children
    a. increased family cohesiveness
    b. joy and happiness
    c. self-enrichment
    d. all of the above

8. What bothers couples most when they become parents?
    a. less money to spend
    b. feeling tired all the time
    c. loss of free time
    d. extra responsibilities

9. Which statement best describes how mothers and fathers view childrearing obligations?
    a. fathers fail to appreciate the everyday life of a mother with small children
    b. fathers tend to choose childrearing tasks they prefer
    c. mothers feel more trapped than fathers because they don't have any one to hand their job to
    d. all of the above are true

10. What do many fathers consider their most important task of the parenting role?
    a. economic support of the family
    b. being supportive of the mother in her duties
    c. sharing in routine child care
    d. spending quality time with his children

11. What conclusion can be drawn about children and stress?
   a. children shouldn't experience stress in their childhood
   b. minimal stress is beneficial in a child's life in order to develop stress tolerance
   c. children should experience a sizable amount of stress because stress is a part of adult life
   d. parent's should deliberately introduce stress into their child's life

12. Research on cultural differences among American ethnic groups has found
   a. ethnic parents tend to be stricter, placing greater demands and expectations on their children
   b. ethnic parents tend to be more lenient on their children due to the hardships they face
   c. there are no cultural differences when to comes to raising children
   d. the research is inconclusive on the differences

13. Studies have found that the _____ parenting style is more likely to produce a competent child.
   a. permissive
   b. overprotective
   c. egalitarian
   d. neglectful

14. Anderson and Collins' review of the literature on television and its effects on children revealed all of the following but one, it is
   a. children are cognitively active while viewing television
   b. children are overstimulated by television
   c. television may actually increase children's attention span
   d. homework done while watching television is not of lower quality than when it is done in silence

15. Which of the following is not one of the three major problems of watching television?
   a. the effects of commercials
   b. the content of programs
   c. the time spent in passive observation
   d. the lack of educational programming

16. Based on the research, what is the relationship between violence on television and later aggressive behavior?
   a. children who watch violence on television are more aggressive in their play
   b. children who watch violence on television are less aggressive in their play
   c. there is no relationship between watching violence and aggression during play
   d. the research is still inconclusive

17. A person who lacks a sense of social responsibility because s/he has not internalized a minimum number of social rules and mores is called a
    a. social misfit
    b. sociologist
    c. sociopath
    d. psychotic

18. High-risk behaviors in parents that may result in a child developing antisocial personality disorder are
    a. minimal touching, stroking, or talking to a baby
    b. not establishing eye contact except when angry
    c. overstimulating the child by talking too much
    d. all of the above

19. What is a predictor of the quality of parenting for both mothers and fathers?
    a. quality of parenting received as a child
    b. education
    c. satisfaction with the parent/child relationship
    d. all of the above

20. On a continuum from mild to strong, which of the following child control methods would be considered at the strong end?
    a. situational assistance
    b. rewarding and contracting
    c. reality and ethical appraisals
    d. supporting the child's self-control

21. In Erikson's stages of psychosocial development, the stage in which children begin to develop self-control and explore and manipulate the environment is
    a. autonomy vs. doubt and shame
    b. initiative vs. guilt
    c. industry vs. inferiority
    d. identity vs. role confusion

22. In Erikson's stages of psychosocial development, the stage in which children broaden their activities, friendships, and achieve more independence is
    a. initiative vs. guilt
    b. autonomy vs. doubt and shame
    c. industry vs. inferiority
    d. trust vs. mistrust

23. The major problem facing parents of teenagers is
    a. drugs
    b. disobedience
    c. giving up control
    d. peer group influence

24. The two major reasons adult children return home to live with their parents are
    a. divorce and needing child care
    b. problems from a divorce and money worries
    c. money problems and needing child care
    d. needing help with raising children and money worries

25. Single-parent families where the woman chooses to become a parent is characterized by all of the following but one:
    a. monetarily successful
    b. have professional careers
    c. are nearing the end of the child-bearing years
    d. have few social resources

Critical Thinking and Decision Making
1. Are we creating sociopaths in this society? Why?
2. Will future generations of children have a more difficult time due to current childrearing practices? Why?
3. Do you want children? Why?
4. Create a list of the pros and cons to having a child. Analyze couples' relationships you know that do and do not have children. How are their lives different?
5. How can a parent combat the negative influences of television?

Examining International Families
1. Discuss the pros and cons to this Kibbutzim way of child rearing.
2. What major adjustments would couples experience if one were reared in a Kibbutz and the other not?

Answers

Key Terms: 1   latchkey children
              2   puberty
              3   adolescence

True/False: 1 T; 2 T; 3 T; 4 T; 5 T; 6 F; 7 T; 8 F; 9 F; 10 F; 11 F; 12 T; 13 T; 14 F

Multiple Choice: 1 b; 2 a; 3 d; 4 c; 5 b; 6 d; 7 d; 8 c; 9 d; 10 a; 11 b; 12 a; 13 c; 14 b; 15 d; 16 a; 17 c; 18 d; 19 d; 20 b; 21 a; 22 c; 23 c; 24 b; 25 d

Chapter 14
Family Life Stages: Middle-Age to Surviving Spouse

Chapter Outline

- Marriage and family relationships change. Change does not mean the end of a relationship. Indeed, lack of change over time is usually unhealthy and may ultimately lead to the demise of the relationship.

Ability to Deal With Change and Stress in a Positive Manner: Another Characteristic of the Strong Family
- Strong families deal with difficulties from a position of strength and solidarity.
- Strong families also remain flexible which helps them weather the storms of life and the inevitable changes that occur.

An Overview of Family Life Stages
- The average American couple goes through six important periods in long-term marriage: _____, early parenthood, _____ , middle-age (empty nest), retirement, and widowed singleness.
- The increase in life expectancy and declining infant mortality has a number of effects on the family:

  _____ .

  . The number of living grandparents is greatly increased for children, and three-, four-, and even five-generation families are more common.
  Marriages potentially can last much longer, so that couples experience middle-age and prolonged retirement together, or they divorce.

  _____ .

  The number of elderly persons depending on middle-aged children is increasing.
  The graying of Americans means that more methods of care for infirm elderly persons must be made available.

- People now spend at least a quarter of their adult lives in retirement. The retiree must cope with a lack of purpose and feelings of uselessness.
- There are about _____ times more widows than widowers in the US.

Middle-Age (The Empty Nest)

- Middle-age starts when children become independent and ends when retirement draws near. Usually between ages 45 and 65 according to the census bureau.
- For most women who have not had a career, adjustment centers on not being needed by their children. For most men, problems center around work and their feelings of achievement and success. Women face their partial failure as parents; men face their failure to achieve all of their dreams.
- Concerns about sexuality arise. Women are concerned with physical attractiveness; men are concerned with performance.
- Middlessence is a term that has been coined for this stage.
- People in middle age find themselves "sandwiched" between young adults who are living with parents longer and longer and aging parents who require care and help.
- In the past young adults, ages 18 to 34, left home earlier with each succeeding generation. In the 1970s the trend began reversing, and now young adults are more likely to be living with their parents. Later marriages, increasing emphasis on education, high housing costs, and higher rates of divorce prompted the reversal.
- Young adults in the home contribute to a high level of parental dissatisfaction. Parents lose privacy, and children may not contribute financially to a share of expenses. Young adults complain about a lack of freedom and parental interference.
- The number of persons over 65 years of age doubled between 1950 and _____ and is predicted to double again by 2050.
- Studies show that daughters and daughters-in-law rather than sons are the primary caregivers to aging parents.
- About _____ percent of Americans in the 50s have older parents in need of care or supervision. Only a small percentage of older parents live in institutions.
- Research suggests that families with younger children still at home have less stress between parents and their older parents for whom they are caring.
- When children are gone, the couple may renew their life together and reinvest in one another.

Retirement

- Retirement age has fallen between four and five years for both men and women since 1950 and is projected to fall even further by 2050.
- Studies about marital satisfaction after retirement are mixed. Some suggest satisfaction increases; some suggest there is little or no relationship between retirement and satisfaction.

- Because retirement comes abruptly for many Americans, it is necessary to prepare ahead, both economically and psychologically. Those who retire optimally maintain activities of middle age as long as possible and then find substitutes for the activities they are forced to give up.
- _____ and _____ seem to be the two most important factors influencing the success of both retirement and general adjustment of old age. Generally, a person's income drops by half upon retirement.

Widowhood as the Last Stage of Marriage

- About 2 percent of women and _____ percent of men over 65 years of age remarry upon losing a spouse, although the percentages seem to be rising.
- Widows seem to have better support systems than widowers (friends, companions, and interaction with children and grandchildren).
- Widowers have higher rates of suicide, physical illness, mental illness, alcoholism, and accidents than widows.
- Studies show no evidence that either men or women are more likely to die in the early months of bereavement.
- _____ by widowers dramatically lowers their mortality rates.
- Mortality rates for both men and women rise dramatically upon moving into a retirement or nursing home, but this is because illness and inability to care for oneself are the usual reasons for making such a move.
- More than _____ of the elderly remain in their home until death. Another 25 percent live with a child.
- About half a million are monetarily able to buy or lease living quarters in exclusive retirement communities.
- The surviving spouse goes through three phases in the grieving process:
    Crisis-loss phase: the survivor is in a state of chaos.
    _____ phase: the survivor attempts to create a new life.
    Establishment and Continuation of a New Lifestyle Phase: a new life or remarriage may occur.
- Most elderly who do remarry report high levels of satisfaction.
- Important questions married people should be able to answer:
    Is there a will? Where is it, and what are its contents?
    Is there life insurance? How much, and how can it be collected?
    What are the financial liabilities and assets?
    Are there safety deposit boxes? Where are the keys?
    How much cash is needed in the next sixty days to keep the family going?

The Grandparenting Role

- Three-quarters of older Americans are grandparents, and of these _____ percent are great grandparents.
- Grandparenting gives people a second chance to be an even better parent and can provide important physical contact.

- Grandparents can become surrogate parents, provide a buffer against family mortality, act as a deterrent against family disruption, and provide a place to go to escape marital difficulties.
- Grandparenting differs by ethnicity and subculture: Latinos and Asian Americans tend to maintain closer relationships between grandparents and grandchildren with Asian-Americans having the highest percentage of relatives living with the parents; a larger percentage of African Americans over 60 years old than whites or Latinos report raising children other than their own.
- All fifty states have statues granting grandparents the right to petition for visits with their grandchildren.
- On the downside, more and more grandparents are missing out on retirement while they serve as surrogate parents.

Older, But Coming on Strong
- Leading a healthy life when young tends to translate into a healthy old age.
- Gerontologist make some strong recommendations for staying healthy longer: _____ ; cut back on drinking; _____ ; avoid foods rich in cholesterol and fat; stress high-fiber foods such as whole grain cereals; and exercise at least three times a week including aerobics and strength training.

Summary
- Families, like people within them, span a long period of time.
- Young families who learn to resolve conflicts and handle the stresses and strains of life will have the best chance of becoming enduring, lasting families.
- When the last child leaves home, the middle-aged (empty nest) stage begins.
- Retirement enters one's thoughts during the middle years. When it finally comes, the family will have adjustments to make.
- Eventually, death must be faced as one spouse (usually, the husband) dies.
- The grandparenting role is taking on more importance as life expectancy increases.

Key Terms
1. When an individual re-evaluates her/his life during the middle-age stage it is referred to as

_____.

True/False Questions
1. _____ In a relationship, the lack of change over time is usually unhealthy and may ultimately lead to the demise of the relationship.
2. _____ Much of the racial difference in life expectancy between black and white populations stems from higher mortality in younger ages.
3. _____ People now spend at least one third of their adult lives in retirement.
4. _____ There are approximately six times more widows than widowers in the United States.

5. _____ Marriage enrichment for the middle-aged couple is not focused so much on improving the marriage as on improving the humans in it.

6. _____ Even though the life span is increasing, Americans can still expect to spend more years caring for their children than they will caring for their parents.

7. _____ Retirement is best characterized as an event rather than a process.

8. _____ Research indicates that the elderly are more prone to hypochondria than the general population.

9. _____ Widowers appear to have better support systems than widows.

10. _____ All fifty states now have statutes granting grandparents the right to petition for visitation with their grandchildren.

Multiple-Choice Questions

1. The stage of a long-term marriage that deals with setting directions for the relationship and learning to work together is the
   a. early parenthood stage
   b. later parenthood stage
   c. newly married stage
   d. middle-age stage

2. The stage of a long-term marriage that deals with the children becoming increasingly independent is the
   a. middle-age stage
   b. later parenthood stage
   c. early parenthood stage
   d. retirement stage

3. Increased life expectancy and declining infant mortality have effected the family in several ways, which is not one of those ways?
   a. children are more likely to know their grandparents
   b. marriages can potentially last longer
   c. more methods of care for the infirmed elderly must be made available
   d. we need two babies to produce one adult

4. The length of retirement has almost doubled in the average worker's life due to what factor?
   a. life expectancy
   b. automation
   c. emphasis on youth
   d. all of the above

5. During middle-age, men's problems usually revolve around
    a. work and their feelings of achievement
    b. money
    c. children
    d. their parents

6. During middle-age, for women who have not had careers, their adjustment usually revolves around
    a. taking care of their parents
    b. dealing with a retiring husband
    c. no longer being needed by their children
    d. social commitments

7. When experiencing menopause, the majority of women report
    a. a decreased interest in sexual activity
    b. an increased interest in sexual activity
    c. no change in their sexual interest
    d. the research is inconclusive at this time

8. For some women, the mid-life crisis may trigger a change in their lives such as
    a. returning to the labor force
    b. entering college
    c. more responsive to competitive feelings
    d. all of the above

9. For men, the mid-life crisis may trigger a change in their lives such as
    a. becoming more interested in family
    b. less responsive to their wives
    c. more interested in work
    d. less interested in social issues

10. Middle-aged parents who are dealing with their children's needs and the needs of aging parents are referred to as
    a. being in a mid-life crisis
    b. the establishment
    c. the sandwich generation
    d. creators of a generation gap

11. What factors contribute to young adult children living with their parents?
    a. divorce
    b. advanced education
    c. cost of living
    d. all of the above

12. Which is not a major complaint of middle-aged parents about having their adult children living at home?
    a. lack of privacy
    b. the friends they bring home
    c. the children's failure to contribute monetarily
    d. sharing in household duties

13. The two main complaints of young adult children living with their parents are
    a. lack of privacy and parental nagging
    b. having to do housework and paying rent
    c. lack of freedom and parental interference
    d. lack of privacy and having to contribute monetarily

14. Who are the primary caregivers of aging parents?
    a. daughters and daughters-in-law
    b. sons and sons-in-law
    c. daughter and sons equally take care of aging parents
    d. adult grandchildren

15. Which statement best describes the relationship between middle-age adults and their parents?
    a. the relationship is a one-way street with adult children taking care of their parents
    b. the relationship is a one-way street with elderly parents taking care of adult children
    c. adult children feel no obligation to take care of their parents
    d. adult children take care of their parents while elderly parents give back to their children by giving advise and/or monetary help

16. Middle-age children are caring for their parents, but who has become known as secondary caregivers?
    a. siblings of the elderly
    b. grandchildren
    c. friends of the elderly
    d. nurses and doctors

17. Which statement best describes the relationship between retirement and marital satisfaction?
    a. marital satisfaction increases after retirement
    b. marital satisfaction decreases after retirement
    c. some studies suggest marital satisfaction increases while other studies find little or no relationship
    d. retirement has no effect on marital satisfaction

18. Which statement best describes who adjusts best to retirement?
    a. those who retire abruptly
    b. those who have prepared economically for retirement
    c. those who are forced to retire due to health problems
    d. those who have prepared economically as well as psychologically by taking on new activities and responsibilities

19. Wives of husbands who have recently retired indicate that the two most positive aspects of his retirement are
    a. time to do what you want and increased companionship
    b. having someone to help with household duties and sharing leisure activities
    c. companionship and having someone to fix things
    d. having someone to share with household duties and increased companionship

20. Wives of husbands who have recently retired indicate that the two most negative aspects of his retirement are
    a. his nagging and his being gone a lot of the time
    b. less time spent together and his unwillingness to share household duties
    c. financial problems and the husband not having enough to do
    d. his friends and financial problems

21. What are the two most important factors influencing the success of both retirement and general adjustment to old age?
    a. education and race
    b. health and money
    c. marital status and race
    d. living arrangements and health

22. What is the retired person's greatest enemy?
    a. taking care of grandchildren
    b. education
    c. ill health
    d. inflation

23. On the average, a women needs to be about _____ years older than her husband to die within one year of each other.
    a. 3
    b. 7
    c. 10
    d. 5

24. The majority of elderly live
    a. with one of their children
    b. in a nursing home
    c. in their own home
    d. with relatives other than children

25. What function can grandparents provide to grandchildren and their families?
    a. arbitrators in family disputes
    b. provide a place to escape marital difficulties
    c. become friends and sometimes allies of their grandchildren
    d. all of the above

Critical Thinking and Decision Making

1. At what age do you think you will retire? Why?
2. What are the pros and cons to having elderly parents live with you and/or your family?
3. What can society do to make life easier for the sandwich generation?
4. How well do you handle stress in your life? What are some of the things you do to relieve stress?
5. What kind of relationship do you have with your parents? Do you think it will change over time? How?
6. What type of relationship do you have with your grandparents? Would you want them living with you? Why?

Answers
Key Terms: 1   middlessence

True/False: 1 T; 2 T; 3 F; 4 T; 5 T; 6 F; 7 F; 8 F; 9 F; 10 T

Multiple-Choice: 1 c; 2 b; 3 d; 4 d; 5 a; 6 c; 7 b; 8 d; 9 a; 10 c; 11 d; 12 b; 13 c; 14 a; 15 d; 16 b; 17 c; 18 d; 19 a; 20 c; 21 b; 22 d; 23 b; 24 c; 25 d

Chapter 15
Family Crises

Chapter Outline

- One of the characteristics of all strong families is the ability to handle crises.
- A crisis is an emotionally significant event or a radical change of status in a person's life. It may involve both negative and positive events: birth of a child, unemployment, moving to a new location, divorce, remarriage, illness, natural catastrophes, injury, and death.
- Whether a change is a crisis depends on the family--its crisis management skills, its resources, and the way it views the turning point.

Coping with Crises
- Stressor events: events that are apt to become crises.
- Husbands are _____ (more or less) likely than wives to bring their home stress into the workplace. Husbands and wives bring work stress home equally.
- Research has found that moderate stress, especially during childhood, may be related to later achievement. Goertzel and Goertzel studied 400 famous men and women of the 20th century and found that three-fourths were troubled as children and that one-fourth had experienced handicaps.
- Individuals exhibit a response to stress called the general-adaptation syndrome consisting of three phases: alarm, resistance, and recovery or exhaustion.
- The steps in crisis management are:
  Describe the event in realistic terms. Determine if it is a crisis for you, your family, or your friend.

  _____ .

  Seek support and help from friends and family who can help you see alternatives.

  _____ .

- Anxiety is a generalized fear without a specific object or source.
- Focusing your energy and relaxing are important when facing a crisis.
- Defense mechanisms used to deny, excuse, change, or disguise behavior that cause anxiety are: repression displacement, _____ , projection, _____ , and _____ .
- Defense mechanisms used in moderate and recognizable manners can contribute to satisfactory adjustments by giving time to adjust to a problem, by leading to experimentation with new roles, and by causing behavior that may be socially useful and even creative.

Death in the Family

- Dying of natural causes, such as old age, may be gradual and expected, and the family can prepare for the death and coming changes. Any sudden death creates an immediate and extremely traumatic shock and crisis for the family.
- The overall homicide rate in the US has dropped from 11 per 100,000 population in the late eighties to 10 per 100,000 in 1992. _____ are six to seven times more likely to die by homicide than whites, dropping from ten times more likely in 1970.
- The overall suicide rate in the US has remained between 10 and 12 per 100,000 for the past fifty years.
- If death comes slowly to a loved one, family members may experience the same basic emotional reactions as the dying person: denial and isolation, _____ , _____ , _____ , and acceptance.
- Many of the same emotional reactions are experienced when facing other crises.
- Grief is natural and is necessary to adjust to the loss of a loved one. At first, there is a period of numbness and shock; followed by pangs of grief, giving way to a prolonged period of dejection and periodic depression. Gradually, life returns to normal.

Accident, Injuries, and Catastrophic Illness

- Statistics show:

    Males have more of every kind of accident than do females for every age after one year.
    People under forty have more accidents than those over forty.

    _____ .
    _____ .

    Most accidental injuries occur in the home.
    Accidental rates peak on certain days such as holidays.
- Several factors increase the chances of accidents: poor physical condition, emotions, and personality traits.
- Because accidents and severe illnesses are unexpected, decision making skills become very important since decisions must be made quickly.

Family Violence

- The number of husbands killing wives and the number of wives killing husbands are about equal.
- Generally, violence flares between spouses who do not have _____ .

- Abuse of husbands by wives most often is _____ rather than physical.
- In a study of singles, cohabitants, and married couples, Stets and Straus found that the most violence occurred among _____ .
- Four elements must be present in a family for child abuse to occur: the parent must be a person to whom physical punishment is acceptable; the abusive parent often has unrealistic expectations for the child; the parent perceives the child to be difficult and trying; and there is usually a crisis of some kind.
- Violence among _____ is the most common form of family violence.
- Factors associated with family violence:
    The cycle of violence
    Socioeconomic status

    _____

    _____

    Traditional male role orientation
    Lack of self-esteem, understanding, patience, and tolerance.

    _____

Poverty and Unemployment
- Most poor families move in and out of poverty depending on family composition and work patterns.
- More than half of the people who are poor live in families with at least one worker.
- The creation of more and better paying jobs and improving education opportunities and standards are two important goals that American society must set if poverty is to be erased.

Drug and Alcohol Abuse
- A drug is any substance _____ .
- Drug abuse is the persistent and excessive use of any drug that results in psychological or physical dependence or which the society labels as dangerous or illegal.
- Physical addiction: a person must use the drug to maintain bodily comfort.
- Drug tolerance: an ever-increasing amount of drug is necessary to maintain comfort.
- Withdrawal symptoms: bodily discomfort that accompanies the discontinued use of a substance.
- _____ is by far America's biggest drug problem.

Summary
- Stress occurs often in everyone's life.
- People usually go through three phases in reacting to stress.
- Successful crisis management involves five steps.
- Death of loved ones is a crisis that all people must face at times in their lives.
- Mourning and grief are natural reactions to a death.
- Sexuality pervades the lives of humans.
- Injuries and prolonged illness can cause lasting changes in family life.

- Family violence can come in many forms: spousal abuse, children abuse, sibling abuse, and parental abuse by children.
- Poverty and unemployment increase the strain on families.
- Drugs and alcohol abuse are contributing factors in many family problems.

Key Terms

1. Any event that provokes a crisis is called a _____.
2. A generalized fear without a specific object or source is called a(n) _____.
3. _____ is when a person deliberately relaxes each muscle in the body starting with the feet and working up to the face.
4. The unconscious blocking of whatever is causing an individual stress or frustration is called _____.
5. The substitution of a less threatening behavior for another is called _____.
6. Finding an excuse for a behavior that is causing trouble is called _____.
7. A defense mechanism where a person imposes their own characteristics or impulses on another person is called _____.
8. The conversion of a socially unacceptable impulse into a socially acceptable activity is called _____.
9. Allowing a person to make up for a shortcoming in one area by becoming successful in another area is called _____.
10. Employed people who live below the poverty threshold are called the _____.
11. Any substance taken for medical purposes or for pleasure that affects bodily functions is called a _____.

True-False Questions

1. _____ Tolerance to stress is a highly individualized response; what is stressful to one may not be stressful to another.
2. _____ As long as a person is in a state of denial, it is impossible to handle a crisis.
3. _____ Crisis management is the ability to make sound decisions and to solve problems constructively.
4. _____ More husbands kill their wives than wives kill their husbands.
5. _____ Abuse of husbands by wives is most often physical rather than verbal.
6. _____ Individuals experiencing spousal violence tend to abuse their children.
7. _____ Research indicates that most people who experience child abuse grow up to abuse others.
8. _____ More male children are sexually molested than female children.
9. _____ One nationally representative study found that child abuse and wife-abuse rates have increased significantly since 1980.
10. _____ More than half of the people who are poor live in families with at least one worker.

Multiple-Choice Questions

1. An event that upsets the smooth functioning of a person's life is called a
     a. transition
     b. crisis
     c. phase
     d. catastrophe

2. Who is more likely to bring home stress into the workplace and work stress into the home?
     a. wives; husbands
     b. husbands; wives
     c. husbands; wives and husbands equally
     d. wives; wives and husbands equally

3. Based on the research, which of the following events is the most stressful?
     a. death of a child
     b. death of a spouse
     c. death of a parent
     d. divorce

4. Which of the following statements is not true about stress?
     a. tolerance to stress varies greatly between people
     b. moderate stress, especially during childhood, may be related to later achievement
     c. some stress in life can be healthful
     d. physical and psychological symptoms to stress are different

5. During general-adaptation-syndrome, the phase in which various physical responses appear to return to normal is
     a. alarm
     b. recovery
     c. resistance
     d. adaptation

6. Methods that an individual uses to deny, excuse, change, or disguise behaviors that cause anxiety are
     a. progressive relaxation techniques
     b. defense mechanisms
     c. crisis management
     d. none of the above

7. Janet loves to play tennis but is not very good, but she studies hard and makes very good grades. This is an example of which defense mechanism?
   a. rationalization
   b. displacement
   c. projection
   d. compensation

8. Nancy missed a deadline at work and told her boss she just had too much work to do. This is an example of which defense mechanism?
   a. rationalization
   b. sublimation
   c. compensation
   d. displacement

9. Which of the following are positive uses of defense mechanisms?
   a. they can give time to adjust to a problem
   b. they may lead to experimentation with new roles
   c. some may be socially useful and even creative
   d. all of the above

10. Who has the highest homicide rate in the US?
   a. Hispanics
   b. Whites
   c. African-Americans
   d. American Indians

11. The stages of dealing with death and dying in order of experience are
   a. anger, denial, bargaining, acceptance, depression
   b. denial, anger, bargaining, depression, acceptance
   c. depression, denial, anger bargaining, acceptance
   d. denial, bargaining, anger, depression, acceptance

12. What is the most common cause of death and injury for young people aged one to twenty-four?
   a. accidents
   b. homicide
   c. suicide
   d. birth defects

13. Statistics show that accidents follow certain patterns. Which is not one of those patterns?
    a. males have more accidents than females
    b. most accidental deaths involve motor vehicles
    c. most accidental injuries occur in the home
    d. most accident victims live in rural areas

14. In general, physical violence flares between spouses who do not have
    a. good sexual relationships
    b. the same value system
    c. good communication skills
    d. the same attitudes about gender roles

15. One study on relationship violence found which group to have the highest rate of violence?
    a. singles
    b. cohabitors
    c. married
    d. separated

16. Which is not one of the elements that must be present in a family for child abuse to occur?
    a. the parent believes physical punishment is acceptable
    b. the parent perceives the child to be difficult and trying
    c. the parent often has realistic expectations for the child
    d. there is usually a crisis of some kind

17. Which is the most common form of family violence?
    a. spousal abuse
    b. child abuse
    c. elderly abuse
    d. sibling abuse

18. Which is not one of the factors associated with family violence?
    a. middle class has the highest rate of violence
    b. social isolation increases the risk that severe violence will occur
    c. abusers and the abused tend to have a low self-esteem
    d. violence begets violence

19. What are two important goals that American society must set if poverty is to be erased in the US?
    a. offer more government programs and improve educational opportunities
    b. create more and better paying jobs and improve educational opportunities and standards
    c. do away with the welfare system and instill a work ethic
    d. create more and better paying jobs and instill a work ethic

20. Which is America's biggest drug problem?
    a. cocaine
    b. alcohol
    c. marijuana
    d. LSD

21. Whether a change is a crisis or not depends on the family's
    a. crisis management skills
    b. resources
    c. way it views the situation
    d. all of the above

22. Which of the following is the major psychological mechanism used in scapegoating?
    a. compensation
    b. sublimation
    c. projection
    d. repression

23. Tools that people use to deal successfully with stressful situations are
    a. assuming responsibility for solving the problem
    b. affirming self-worth
    c. balance self-concern with other-concern
    d. all of the above

24. Which is not one of the causes of attempted suicide?
    a. they may be trying to get attention
    b. they have a realistic view of death
    c. they may have a parent or friend who committed suicide
    d. they may be under the influence of drugs

25. The stage of death and dying in which one questions why this is happening is
    a. anger
    b. denial
    c. bargaining
    d. depression

Critical Thinking and Decision Making
1. What are ways that you handle stress in your life?
2. Why do you think alcohol is our major drug problem in the US? What should we do to combat this?
3. Have you ever considered suicide? What prompted you to think about this alternative?
4. Have you ever been the victim of abuse? What did you do about this situation?
5. How should society attack the issue of poverty? What effects does this have on individuals and families?

Answers

Key Terms: 1   stressor event
              2   anxiety
              3   progressive relaxation
              4   repression
              5   displacement
              6   rationalization
              7   projection
              8   sublimation
              9   compensation
              10   working poor
              11   drug

True-False: 1 T; 2 T; 3 T; 4 F; 5 F; 6 T; 7 F; 8 F; 9 F; 10 T

Multiple Choice: 1 b; 2 c; 3 a; 4 d; 5 c; 6 b; 7 d; 8 a; 9 d; 10 c; 11 b; 12 a; 13 d; 14 c; 15 b; 16 c; 17 d; 18 a; 19 b; 20 b; 21 d; 22 c; 23 d; 24 b; 25 a

Chapter 16
The Dissolution of Marriage

Chapter Outline

<u>Let No One Put Asunder</u>
- In the past, a good marriage was measured by how well each spouse fulfilled socially prescribed roles. Today Americans ask a great deal more of marriage, and the higher the stakes, the higher the chances of failure.
- The divorce rate: in 1900, one in twelve marriages; in 1922, one in eight; in the late 1940s, one in three & a half; and in 1984, one in two. Today, the median duration of marriage until divorce is about seven years.
- Crude divorce rate: ratio of divorces to each thousand persons in a population. It varies between 4.6 and 4.9.
- _Serial_ marriages: America's tendency to marry, divorce, and remarry.
- Marriage rates are _higher_ (higher or lower) for divorced persons than for single persons.

<u>Reasons for America's High Divorce Rate</u>
- Reasons for the high divorce rate in America:
    Personal reasons such as lack of communication, sexual failure, or overuse of alcohol.
    High expectations often lead to disappointment and failure.
    The relative freedom to make marital choices.
    Changing gender roles in the concept of change & its benefits
    Greater economic indep. of wom. encourages separation & divorce
    Heterogeneity - marriage means different things to people
    Mobility of Americans.

Social upheaval, economic problems, and the general health of society.
Acceptance of divorce.
Personal inadequacies, failures and problems.

Emotional Divorce and the Emotions of Divorce
- Almost always, one of the partners is the initiator who unilaterally begins the uncoupling process, consciously or unconsciously. The initiator gradually withdraws from the relationship and begins to build a new world for him or herself--often unknowingly to the partner.
- Wallerstein and Blakeslee found that only 10 percent of divorced couples were able to construct happier, fuller lives for both husband and wife by the tenth year after the divorce.
- The peak year for breakups of marriage is the _3rd_ year; however, 40 percent of all broken marriages last ten or more years.
- During divorce, most persons will go through a period of denial followed by grief, mourning, and a mixture of self-pity, vengeance, despair, wounded pride, anguish, guilt, loneliness, fear, distrust, withdrawal, relief, and loss of feelings of psychological well-being.
- During separation panic, most people experience _it is an apprehensiveness or anxiety_
- Wallerstein and Blakeslee found that the hurt, hostility, and anger don't disappear even after ten to fifteen years, especially for children.

Divorce But Not the End of the Relationship
- Divorced people often remain bound to one another by children, love, hate, revenge, friendship, business matters, dependence, moral obligations, the need to dominate or rescue, or habit.
- Increasingly, divorce does not dissolve a family unit but simply changes its nature, especially for children.
- The best divorce adjustment is probably attained in an "amicable divorce".

Problems of the Newly Divorced
- Newly divorced person face several major dangers:
     Making a prolonged retreat from social contact.
     May jump quickly into a new marriage
     They base life on the hope that the spouse will return.
     Organizing their life around hostility and getting even.
- Community divorce refers to the effect on the divorcing couple's friends, extended families, and their workplace.
- Most divorced people start to date within the first year after their separation.
- Divorced _Men_ experience a rise in their standard of living in the first year after divorce, while divorced _Women_ and their children experience a decline.
- Only about 60 to 70 percent of mothers are awarded child support. Only about 50 percent of the mothers due support actually receive the full amount from their husbands.

- The trend toward " ~~child support~~ *no fault* " divorce has tended to reduce alimony awards. Only 50 to 75 percent of women awarded alimony receive the full amount from their husbands.
- State, local, and federal governments have tried to strengthen laws to enforce child support and alimony payments.
- The effects of divorce on children is not understood. The immediate effect, usually negative, varies from child to child.
- Wallerstein found that about a quarter of the adults and children experiencing a divorce are resilient, about a half muddle through, and the remaining quarter fail to recover.
- Children who adjusted well to a divorce are those who have strong, well-integrated personalities and those where both parents continue to be part of the children's' lives.
- Boys typically have _*more*_ (more or less) difficulty in adjusting to divorce than girls.
- Courts have four choices in awarding custody of children:
    *Sole* ~~custody~~ custody to one parent (65 to 70 percent). Of these the mother is awarded custody 88 percent of the time.
    *joint* custody in which time is divide with both parents.
    *Split* custody in which the custody of individual children is split between parents.
    Custody to someone other than the parents.

Divorce: The Legalities

- Matrimonial law is one of the most dynamic in the country today.
- Divorce is regulated by state law.
- Since the 1960s, most states have passed laws allowing "no-fault" divorces in which either party was not blamed for the divorce. Irreconcilable differences, mutual consent, or living apart for a time period are sufficient reasons for such divorces. If the parties to the divorce agree and have divided their community property evenly, the courts do not involve themselves in property settlements. Rehabilitative alimony is usually granted to the wife for time periods that generally increase the longer the marriage has existed.
- Reviewable alimony can be extended beyond the end of the limited term if the need still exists.
- A new "do-it-yourself" trend in divorce has developed that does not require the use of attorneys. The parties go directly to the courts and obtain divorces for the cost of filing ($100 to $400).
- Problems with no-fault divorces include:
    They generally cause a severe economic hardship on divorced women and their children.
    Property settlements may be incomplete or grossly unfair to one of the pair.
    The reduction of majority age from 21 to 18 means custodial parents carry a heavier burden earlier to support children.
- _____ provides a setting in which the couple can meet, communicate, and negotiate a settlement with professional help to present to the court.
- _____ occurs after the divorce is final and is aimed at helping the individuals get life started again.

Reducing Divorce Rates
* Steps that might reduce the divorce rate:
    More effective marriage and family training.

    _____ .

    _____ .

    Laws to encourage couples to take marriage more seriously.

    _____ .

    Giving at least as much attention to the positive aspects of marriage as we do to the negative aspects.

Divorce May Not Be The Answer
* More and more family counselors are finding that the problems surrounding a divorce are far worse than the problems within the marriage. Therefore, more counselors are working to help solve marital problems rather than helping face the problems of divorce.

Summary
* The divorce rate has increased drastically during this century, probably reflecting Americans' changing expectations for marriage and increasing tolerance of change.
* There are many reasons for the high divorce rate in the United States.
* The decision to divorce is usually reached slowly and involves emotions similar to the feelings that one goes through after the death of a loved one.
* Divorced people must cope with numerous problems.
* In the past few years, all states have instituted some form of no-fault divorces.

Key Terms
1. The __Crude divorce rate__ is the ratio of divorces to each thousand person within the population.
2. __Serial marriages__ refers to individuals who marry, divorce, and remarry.
3. Divorce proceedings that do not place blame for the divorce on one spouse or the other is called a __No fault Divorce__ .
4. An award of alimony that is reviewed periodically and changed if necessary is called __Reotewable Alimony__ .
5. The taking of children from the custodial parent by the noncustodial parent after a divorce is called __child snatching__ .

True-False Questions

1. __T__ The partner who has the power in the breakup process is the one who initiated the divorce.
2. __F__ Girls typically show more maladjustment and more prolonged problems than boys.
3. __T__ In the past, payment of alimony was sometimes used to punish the guilty spouse rather than to help a spouse become reestablished.
4. __T__ Couples who can work out their differences before going to court are in a better position to obtain a fair and equitable divorce.
5. __F__ Research upheld the popular belief that easier divorce laws would lead to skyrocketing divorce rates.
6. __T__ Because children are seen as adults at the age of 18 and child support payments stop, many children of divorce have difficulty obtaining a postsecondary degree.
7. __T__ More and more family counselors are discovering that the problems surrounding the divorce are often far worse than the problems within the marriage.
8. __T__ The better the couple's communication and understanding, the less traumatic the divorce will be, both for themselves and for any children they may have.
9. __F__ With alimony and child support payments, divorced women experience a rise in their standard of living in the first year after divorce, while divorced men experience a decline.
10. __F__ Joint custody is more prevalent among whites and those who have higher income and educational levels.
11. __T__ Some people advocate that rather than trying to maintain marriage through strict divorce laws, a better approach might be to make marriages harder to enter.
12. __F__ Divorce mediation occurs after the divorce is final and is aimed at helping the individuals get life started again.

Multiple-Choice Questions

1. Today, the medium duration of marriage until a divorce is approximately
   a. 5 years
   b. 3 years
   c. 7 years
   d. 10 years

2. Which of the following is an example of one who engages in serial marriages?
   a. Elizabeth Taylor
   b. George Bush
   c. Bill Clinton
   d. Al Gore

3. Which is not one of the reasons for America's high divorce rate?
    a. we ask a great deal of modern marriages
    b. we tend to marry people with similar backgrounds
    c. greater economic independence of women
    d. changing gender roles

4. Marital failure is highest among the
    a. upper class
    b. middle class
    c. lower class
    d. homeless

5. In the divorce process outlined in the chapter, in which stage will the emotional stress be the greatest?
    a. when the possibility of divorce is first mentioned
    b. when they are actually divorced
    c. when they have made the decision to divorce
    d. when they physically separate

6. In Bohannan's stations of divorce, the station that deals with the property settlement is the
    a. community divorce
    b. economic divorce
    c. legal divorce
    d. psychological divorce

7. In Bohannan's stations of divorce, the station dealing with the reactions of friends and extended family is
    a. community divorce
    b. parental divorce
    c. emotional divorce
    d. psychological divorce

8. In Bohannan's stations of divorce, the station that many consider to be the most important is the
    a. emotional divorce
    b. parental divorce
    c. psychological divorce
    d. economic divorce

9. The initiator of a divorce
     a. often begins the process of withdrawing from the relationship
     b. has the power in the relationship
     c. is more likely to view the divorce as positive
     d. all of the above

10. Which is not one of the major dangers for the newly divorced person?
     a. they retreat from social contact for too long
     b. they want to totally forget the ex-spouse
     c. they hope that the spouse will return
     d. they jump quickly into a new marriage

11. Remaining friends with a newly divorced person is difficult for all but one of the following reasons, it is
     a. the divorce causes the couple's married friends to reexamine their own marriages
     b. the married friends may experience conflict about which partner will remain a friend
     c. married friends feel an obligation to find dating partners for the newly divorced person
     d. the married friends may view the newly single person as a threat to their relationship

12. Approximately _____ of the mothers due court-ordered support from their children's father actually receive the full amount.
     a. half
     b. one-fourth
     c. three-fourths
     d. two-thirds

13. Child support is based on
     a. mother's income at the time of the divorce
     b. the children's needs and the parents ability to pay
     c. the overall divorce settlement
     d. mother's income and the children's needs

14. Combining unmarried birth with the current rate of divorce, about _____ percent of children born today will likely spend some of their childhood in a single-parent family.
     a. 50
     b. 25
     c. 60
     d. 75

15. Guidelines for telling children about an impending divorce include
    a. do not place blame on a partner
    b. both parents telling the children
    c. describing some of your attempts to protect and improve the marriage
    d. all of the above

16. In Wallerstein's study of sixty families going through a divorce, she found
    a. the great majority adjusted successfully
    b. three-fourths were either muddling through or failing to recover
    c. half adjusted successfully and half were muddling through
    d. ninety percent were failing to recover and looking back with intense longing

17. According to Wallerstein's study, the children who made the best adjustments to the divorce were those who
    a. had a good sense of humor
    b. could see both sides of the divorce
    c. had well-integrated and adjusted personalities
    d. had strong relationships with both their parents

18. Research indicates that fatherless children are more vulnerable to
    a. poverty
    b. drugs
    c. school failure
    d. all of the above

19. Which age group is more likely to blame themselves for the divorce?
    a. preschoolers
    b. seven and eight year olds
    c. adolescents
    d. nine to ten year olds

20. Which age group is more likely to experience a conflict of loyalty?
    a. preschoolers
    b. nine to ten year olds
    c. adolescents
    d. seven to eight year olds

21. Who are the forgotten victims of divorce?
    a. friends
    b. cousins
    c. grandparents
    d. aunts and uncles

22. What two factors must be considered in understanding the effects of divorce on children?
    a. who gets custody and the sex of the children
    b. age and sex of the child
    c. age of the child and their support networks
    d. none of the above

23. The custody arrangement in which the children divide their time between the parents is called
    a. joint custody
    b. sole custody
    c. split custody
    d. guardian custody

24. Which of the following is not one of the factors in noncustodial fathers' failure to visit their children?
    a. conflict with the ex-spouse
    b. guilt over nonpayment of support
    c. having a new family
    d. living near the children

25. The do-it-yourself approach to divorce is not recommended unless
    a. the partners are relatively friendly
    b. they agree on all matters
    c. they do not have a large income, assets, or liabilities
    d. all of the above

Critical Thinking and Decision Making

1. Do you think laws should be stricter or more lenient with regards to divorce? Why?
2. What are the pros and cons to the different types of child custody arrangements?
3. What do you think the American society should do to lower the divorce rate?
4. What should be done to encourage fathers to maintain contact with their children after divorce and to continue child support payments?
5. In your opinion, why is the divorce rate so high in the US?

Answers

Key Terms: 1   crude divorce rate
            2   serial marriages
            3   no fault divorce
            4   reviewable alimony
            5   child snatching

True/False: 1 T; 2 F; 3 T; 4 T; 5 F; 6 T; 7 T; 8 T; 9 F; 10 F; 11 T; 12 F

Multiple Choice: 1 c; 2 a; 3 b; 4 c; 5 d; 6 b; 7 a; 8 c; 9 d; 10 b; 11 c; 12 a; 13 b; 14 c; 15 c; 16 b; 17 c; 18 d; 19 a; 20 b; 21 c; 22 b; 23 a; 24 d; 25 d

Chapter 17
Remarriage: A Growing Way of American Life

Chapter Outline

- Approximately 50 percent of marriages are remarriages.
- Originally *step* in *stepfather, stepmother,* and *stepfamily,* meant "_____". Most of today's stepchildren have both biological parents.
- Age differences between remarried spouses tend to be greater than between first-married couples (four years versus two years). For remarriages of never-married women and divorced men, the average age difference is seven years.
- _____ monogamy: several spouses over a lifetime but only one at a time.

Returning to Single Life
- The return to single life can be frightening for both men and women. Most people have experienced a blow to their self-esteem with the divorce and are reluctant to face potential rejection.
- The newly divorced, especially a person who has been rejected by a spouse, may initially engage in sexual experimentation to boost their shattered self-esteem. They must guard against sexual exploitation.
- Legitimate classified ads are increasingly being used by divorced persons to seek desirable companions and potential mates.
- Computer and video dating are also used to meet new persons but at considerable expense.
- The most important step the newly divorced can take is to participate actively in the singles' world.
- Despite the additional problems children create for the dating divorced parent, most research shows that children do not reduce the chances for remarriage.
- Dating divorced persons differ from the single dating person in _____ , _____ , and _____ .
- Divorced people tend to marry _____ (divorced or single) people.

- Divorced men tend to remarry _____ (more or less) quickly and at a higher rate than divorced women.
- Divorce women who are older, highly educated, and financially independent are less likely to remarry.
- While cohabitation among never-married young persons appears to have a negative relationship to later marital success, divorced persons who cohabit seem to increase their chances of success in a remarriage.
- Ganong and Coleman found that 59 percent of divorced persons cohabited before remarriage.

Remarriage: Will I Make the Same Mistakes Again?
- Some divorced persons marry a transition person: a person who out of friendship and sympathy has helped through a difficult period such as a divorce.
- Most divorced persons believe that they were deluded in their first marriage and therefore approach a second marriage with extra care.
- Partners in remarriage must face the same problems of the newly married; in addition, they must deal with attitudes and sensitivities within themselves that were fostered by the first marriage.
- Remarriage between divorced persons is more difficult than a first marriage because:
    Each mate may have problems of low self-esteem stemming from the divorce.

    _____ .

    _____ .

    Remarriages involving children will experience many more complications.
    The society around the remarrying person tends to expect another failure.
- Remarried couples indicate money and children are their two major problems as well as the top two reasons for remarriage failure.
- The average child is _____ years old at the time parents divorce.
- Most studies show that a remarriage is more likely to break up than a first marriage, but the differences are small and do not take into account the small group of divorce-prone people who marry and divorce often.
- Remarriages of divorced persons that do not end quickly in divorce are generally as successful as intact first marriages.
- The division of labor in remarriage tends to be more equitable.
- Though the statistics are mixed on the success of remarriages, it is clear that a great many are successful despite the extra problems involved.

His, Hers, and Ours: The Stepfamily
- For couples divorcing from a first marriage, 61 percent had children under 18 years old.
- Having custody of children does not seem to influence one's chances of remarriage. Remarriages often involve three sets of children: the children each spouse brings into the marriage and children they may have together.
- Blended family: the new family of divorced persons, including children.
- Eighty-two percent of remarriages are stepfather families.

- Ganong and Coleman found that stepfathers seem to have an _____ (harder or easier) time with stepchildren than do stepmothers.
- About half of the women who remarry give birth in their second marriage, most within 24 months of remarriage.
- Ganong and Coleman found that a new child can be a source of integration in a stepfamily because everyone finally has someone to whom all are related.
- Research shows that opposite-sex stepsiblings tend to be sexually involved with each other much more frequently than opposite-sex biological siblings.

The New Extended Family
- The immediate effect of divorce on relative interaction is that it intensifies contacts between blood relatives and curtails relations with former in-laws.
- To a large extent, it is up to the various parties involved to determine the extent to which potential kin will be treated as actual relatives.

Building Stepfamily Strengths
- There is little empirical evidence to support the supposed advantages about stepfamilies cited in popular literature.
- A prenuptial agreement is more important in a remarriage than in a first marriage since _____ and _____ are the two major sources of conflict in a remarriage.
- Although few remarrying couples consult mediators or counselors before they marry, such an experience is demonstrably worthwhile.
- By using the wealth of knowledge and experience each new spouse brings to a remarriage, the couple can create a strong and healthy new family.

Summary
- High remarriage rates indicate that the high divorce rates do not necessarily mean that Americans are disenchanted with marriage as an institution.
- The majority of divorced persons remarry, most of them within a few years of divorce.
- People marrying for a second time carry with them attitudes and expectations from their first marital experience.
- Children from prior marriages often add to the responsibilities of second marriage.
- About 20 to 30 percent of those divorcing never remarry.

Key Terms

1. Being married and divorced several times throughout one's lifetime is known as _Serial monogamy_.
2. The spouse of one of your biological parents is known as a _Stepparent_.

True-False Questions

1. __T__ Age differences between remarried spouses tend to be greater than between first-married couples.
2. __T__ Those who have been left against their will are more likely to find single life more difficult than those who have voluntarily left their marriage.
3. __F__ Most of the research indicates that children reduce the chances for remarriage.
4. __F__ Divorced people tend to marry people who have never been married.
5. __F__ Divorced women tend to remarry more quickly and at a higher rate than divorced men.
6. __F__ The research indicates that the wicked stepmother as portrayed in fairy tales is a true description of stepmothers today.
7. __F__ Most research indicates that stepmothers seem to have an easier time with stepchildren than do stepfathers.
8. __T__ The longer a family is a single-parent family, the harder the adjustment will be for the children to the new stepparent.
9. __T__ Conflict is more likely in a remarriage than in a first marriage.
10. __T__ The majority of divorced persons remarry, most of them within a few years of divorce.

Multiple-Choice Questions

1. What is the percentage of divorced men and women that remarry?
   a. 4 out of 5 men and 3 out of 4 women
   b. 3 out of 4 men and 2 out of 5 women
   c. 3 out of 5 men and 2 out of 5 women
   d. 3 out of 4 men and 4 out of 5 women

2. Which racial group has the highest rate of remarriage?
   a. African-American
   b. Asian
   c. Whites
   d. Hispanic

3. What do couples in May-December marriages report about their marital satisfaction?
    a. they report lower levels of marital satisfaction
    b. they report higher levels of marital satisfaction
    c. their marital satisfaction is about the same as other marriages
    d. the research is inconclusive

4. Most people take approximately _____ year(s) to recover emotionally from a divorce.
    a. 2
    b. 1
    c. 3
    d. 4

5. Which is not one of the differences between the divorced dating person and the single dating person?
    a. the divorced person will be older
    b. the divorced person is likely to have children
    c. the divorced person is more knowledgeable about marriage
    d. the divorced person is less likely to have a job

6. Which group remarries more quickly?
    a. women who are less educated and have lower incomes
    b. men who are less educated and have lower incomes
    c. women who are older, highly educated, and financially independent
    d. none of the above

7. Research on cohabitation among never-married young persons indicates what about their later marital success?
    a. they are more likely to stay married
    b. they are more likely to divorce
    c. it has no effect on martial success
    d. b and c are correct

8. The most common reaction of people contemplating remarriage is
    a. to move quickly to alleviate the loneliness
    b. they take about the same amount of time as they did the first time
    c. they tend to be more careful, cautious, and slower to act
    d. the research is inconclusive

9. Partners in a remarriage must deal with all of the following but one.
   a. inappropriate attitudes and behaviors stemming from the first marriage
   b. a lack of trust in others
   c. prejudices for and against marriage
   d. attitudes and sensitivities within themselves that were fostered by the first marriage

10. A remarriage between divorced persons is more difficult than a first marriage because
    a. of past spouses
    b. lower self-esteems stemming from the divorce
    c. they are less likely to tolerate a poor second marriage
    d. all of the above

11. What are the top two reasons people give for failure of their remarriages?
    a. money and children
    b. discipline of children and ex-spousal interference
    c. money and frequency of sex
    d. in-laws and children

12. Of the steps individuals can take to help their chances of remarriage success, the one most often used is
    a. counseling
    b. support groups
    c. reading self-help materials and books
    d. attending seminars

13. Studies indicate that _____ percent of remarriages end in divorce.
    a. 50
    b. 60
    c. 30
    d. 45

14. Studies on marital satisfaction show all of the following but one.
    a. women tend to be more satisfied than men with their remarriages
    b. men tend to be more satisfied than women with their remarriages
    c. stepfathers and stepmothers indicate about the same level of remarriage satisfaction
    d. people in first marriages report greater marital satisfaction than those in remarriages

15. Couples in remarriages state that their remarriage is better than their first marriage because
    a. they have chosen a better mate
    b. they have learned how to communicate differently
    c. they have learned how to handle conflict more maturely
    d. all of the above

16. Overall, research findings on the effects of remarriage on children indicates
    a. children in stepfamilies do better than in their original families
    b. children in stepfamilies do worse than in their original families
    c. children aren't any better off in the second family than in the first
    d. the research findings are mixed

17. Therapists report that stepchildren and stepparents have a great deal of trouble in their new relationships, which of the following is true:
    a. stepparents often feel confused about their roles
    b. children feel loyalty conflicts
    c. coparenting of children with former spouses may split parental authority
    d. all of the above are true

18. Probably the single most important thing divorcing parents can do to reduce the negative consequences of divorce and remarriage on their children is
    a. talk with the child about problems in the marriage
    b. maintain a reasonable relationship with the divorced mate
    c. encourage contact with the other parent
    d. maintain regular schedule and routine

19. Guidelines for surviving as a stepparent include
    a. not expecting instant love
    b. don't try to fit a preconceived role
    c. expect ambivalence from stepchildren
    d. all of the above

20. All but one are things a stepparent can do to help the stepfamily adjust, it is
    a. set limits and enforce them
    b. place some responsibility on the child for making this relationship work
    c. try to keep the children in their original home
    d. be patient with the children

21. Approximately what percent of women who remarry give birth in their second marriage?
    a. 70
    b. 50
    c. 40
    d. 30

22. What things can a stepparent bring to the stepparent-stepchild relationship?
    a. love
    b. support
    c. friendship
    d. all of the above

23. Who reports more stress, dread, and ambivalent feelings about stepchildren?
    a. nonresidential stepmothers
    b. custodial stepmothers
    c. custodial stepfathers
    d. all of the above

24. Belovitch suggests a number of helpful hints for weekend visits, which is not one of them?
    a. give the child a permanent place to store some things
    b. spend time alone with each child
    c. don't allow the child to bring a friend for the weekend as it takes time away from you
    d. establish consistent routines or chores to do

25. Because remarriages are more complicated and difficult than first marriages, the author suggests what as one of the best ways to build a healthy stepfamily?
    a. allow the child to have their way at first
    b. cultivate a sense of humor
    c. spend some time alone with the child
    d. encourage the biological parent to spend more time with their children

Critical Thinking and Decision Making
1. What do you see as the hardest thing about getting along with stepparents?
2. If remarriages are so difficult, should we discourage people from remarrying? Why?
3. What are the advantages and disadvantages to divorce for the couple as well as the children?
4. Compare and contrast dating as a never married person with dating as a divorced person.
5. What are the pros and cons to a prenuptial agreement for people who are remarrying?

Answers

Key Terms: 1   serial monogamy
              2   stepparent

True/False: 1 T; 2 T; 3 F; 4 F; 5 F; 6 F; 7 F; 8 T; 9 T; 10 T

Multiple Choice: 1 a; 2 c; 3 b; 4 b; 5 d; 6 a; 7 d; 8 c; 9 b; 10 d; 11 a; 12 c; 13 b; 14 a; 15 d; 16 d; 17 d; 18 b; 19 d; 20 c; 21 b; 22 d; 23 a; 24 c; 25 b

Chapter 18
Actively Seeking Marital Growth and Fulfillment

Chapter Outline

- Every person has the ability to improve his or her marriage.

<u>"And They Lived Happily Ever After"</u>
- A number of factors combine to keep Americans from working to improve their marriage:
    Myth of naturalism: marriage is "natural" and takes care of itself if we select the right partner.
    _____ : it's bad taste to reveal our intimate and personal lives publicly.
    _____ : treating marriage as a joke and heading off attempts to improve it.
- In order to improve a marriage, it is first necessary to believe it is possible.
- To improve a marriage, couples must work on three things: _____ , their relationship, and the economic environment within which the marriage exists.

<u>Marriage Improvement Programs</u>
- Help for families in the past usually came from relatives, friends, ministers, and family doctors.
- Marital improvement techniques today include:

Courses on marriage and the family	Encounter groups
Family enrichment weekends	Women's and men's consciousness raising groups
Psychodrama	Married couples' communication workshops
Message and bodily awareness training	Sensitivity training
Sex therapy and sexuality workshops	Marriage counseling and family service organizations

- Things a couple can do to improve their relationship:

  _____ .

  Read self-improvement books together, books that discuss relationships, or other books of mutual interest.

  Go out on a "date" often and do things you both like, things that are romantic, or things that bring back happy memories.

  _____ .

- _____ : a focus on your internal sensory, thinking, and emotional processes.
- Partner awareness: knowing accurately what your partner is experiencing in terms of his or her self-awareness.
- _____ : focuses on the interactional patterns of the couple or the entire family.
- Topical awareness: encompasses references to events, objects, ideas, places, and people.

Marriage with Purpose: Effective Management

- Work, leisure, economics, emotions, interests, sex, children, eating, and maintaining the household all require effective management in the fully functioning family.

The Family Will Remain and Diversify

- The family has always been with us and always will be, and it will always change.
- The following might help the family to better meet the challenges of the 1990s:

  _____ .

  Family life education must begin early and train young people in the art of healthy marital communication and family relationships.

  The image of marriage and family conveyed in the popular culture and media needs to be improved.

- Survivors (those who face and solve problems):

  Have insight into themselves and the world in which they live.

  Are able to take the initiative and take charge of their problems rather than only reacting to the challenges of life.

  Have a core set of values and beliefs to sustain them and direct their behavior under adversity.

  Have a humor that can find the comic in the tragic, that can make them laugh at their own mistakes and shortcomings, and remind them that the joy in life most often resides within rather than without.

Summary

- The newly married couple must commit themselves to the idea of working not only to maintain but also to improve their relationship.
- Unfortunately, a number of factors work against such commitment to improve a relationship.
- To improve an intimate relationship, a couple must work on three things: themselves as individuals, their relationship, and the economic environment within which their relationship exists.
- There are now many marriage improvement programs from which couples may choose.

- Marriage and family enrichment programs are aimed at families that do not have serious problems.
- As unromantic as it may sound, a fulfilling marriage and family life is largely based on good management.
- The flexible nature of the family allows it to survive as the major institution for intimate decisions.

Key Terms

1. The idea that marriage is "natural" and will take care of itself if we just choose the right partner is called the _____.
2. The belief that marriage and family life are private and not to be discussed publicly is called

_____.

True-False Questions

1. _____ Marriage is an end result, not a process.
2. _____ Rather than viewing differences and conflicts as signs of incompatibility, couples need to see them as opportunities for growth.
3. _____ Criteria used to judge marriages have shifted from how well members fulfill roles and perform marital functions to whether partners have achieved personal fulfillment and happiness.
4. _____ A successful family is able to find a balance between personal freedom and happiness, and family support and togetherness.
5. _____ Marriage and family enrichment programs are aimed at families that have serious problems.
6. _____ If people spent as much time working on their marriages as they do seeking an ideal alternative, their marriages might be better.
7. _____ Individuals in relationships can never emphasize self-fulfillment and human growth too much.
8. _____ One purpose of marriage enrichment programs is to help couples and families develop a plan for handling disputes and conflicts.
9. _____ A fulfilling marriage and family life is largely based on good management.
10. _____ The author of the text believes the family will not die but will always be with us.

Multiple-Choice Questions

1. A central theme for every couple's marriage should be
    a. dealing with life on a day to day basis
    b. helping each other change
    c. finding ways to revitalize a marriage
    d. finding self-fulfillment

2. Marriages tend to get into trouble because
    a. they believe they can't do much about their marriage
    b. they don't take time to make the relationship healthier
    c. security and comfort lull us into avoiding risks
    d. all of the above

3. Which is not one of the characteristics of a strong, successful family?
    a. appreciation of all family members
    b. dealing with problems only when they arise
    c. good communication
    d. spending time together

4. Which is not one of the factors that keeps most Americans from working actively to improve their marriages?
    a. the principle of least interest
    b. the myth of naturalism
    c. privatism
    d. cynicism

5. The idea that our personal lives are no one's business but our own is an example of
    a. the myth of naturalism
    b. privatism
    c. cynicism
    d. family values

6. "You should have known better than to get married. Don't complain to me about your problems." is an example of
    a. privatism
    b. the myth of naturalism
    c. cynicism
    d. negativity

7. To improve an intimate relationship, couples should work on all of the following but one.
    a. having children
    b. themselves as individuals
    c. their relationship
    d. the economic environment in which their relationship exists

8. More and more family researchers as well as general observers of American society see
   _____ as America's greatest enemy.
   a. personal fulfillment
   b. excessive hedonism
   c. money
   d. none of the above

9. Overall, the major point of this chapter is
   a. greed can destroy everything
   b. people are too concerned about themselves
   c. effective family relationships don't just happen, you have to work at them
   d. if we don't act know, families will be a dying breed

10. Traditionally, marriage was an institution for
    a. childrearing
    b. economic support
    c. proper fulfillment of marital duties
    d. all of the above

11. Due to what factor have the lifestyles of most American families moved slowly toward separate
    conjugal relationships?
    a. the entry of wives in the labor force
    b. the women's liberation movement
    c. social support for individual growth and fulfillment
    d. all of the above

12. Groups that confront a person, forcing him/her to examine problems are called
    a. family enrichment weekends
    b. psychodrama
    c. encounter groups
    d. consciousness raising groups

13. Groups where individuals engage in exercises such as touching, concentrating, heightening awareness,
    and empathizing with one's mate are called
    a. psychodrama
    b. sensitivity training
    c. massage and bodily awareness training
    d. sex therapy and sexuality workshops

14. Groups where couples learn how to fight fairly and engage in role playing are called
    a. married couples' communication workshops
    b. family enrichment weekends
    c. encounter groups
    d. marriage counseling

15. Courses aimed at helping people better understand the institution of marriage are called
    a. encounter groups
    b. family enrichment weekends
    c. marriage and family courses
    d. consciousness raising groups

16. Couples who are not willing to seek outside help can engage in several practices on their own, one of which is
    a. set aside scheduled times each week to talk
    b. read books together on self-improvement or building relationships
    c. go out on a date
    d. all of the above

17. Which is not one of the possible negative effects of the Marriage Encounter program?
    a. perceived benefits may be temporary at best
    b. stress on the relationship may tend to focus on individual differences
    c. communication techniques taught may make the couple's communication patterns more rigid
    d. there may be a divisive influences on the couple's relationship with other family members

18. When choosing a marriage enrichment activity, couples should follow some guidelines, they are
    a. participate together if possible
    b. never get into a group experience on impulse
    c. don't remain in a group that has an ax to grind
    d. all the above

19. The goal of marriage enrichment programs is to
    a. help good marriages be even better
    b. keep the couple from divorcing
    c. encourage self-fulfillment
    d. look at weaknesses of the relationship

20. Components of a marriage enrichment program are
    a. enhancing the couple's communication and emotional life
    b. enhancing the sexual relationship
    c. fostering marriage strengths
    d. all of the above

21. The purpose of family life enrichment programs is to
    a. make the marital relationship better
    b. help families with severe problems
    c. strengthen the marriage as well as the entire family
    d. help siblings get along better

22. Of the four subcategories of marriage enrichment, the one that focuses on internal sensory, thinking, and emotional processes is
    a. relationship awareness
    b. self-awareness
    c. partner awareness
    d. topical awareness

23. Effective management helps families
    a. run smoothly and achieve goals
    b. reduce frustrations and conflicts
    c. maintain flexibility needed to cope with unforeseen emergencies
    d. all of the above

24. Suggestions to help the family meet the challenges of the 1990's include
    a. creating a workplace that is "family friendly"
    b. starting family life training at an early age
    c. improve the media's portrayal of marriages and families
    d. all of the above

25. Which of the following is a characteristic of a survivor?
    a. they have insight into themselves and the world
    b. they take charge of their problems
    c. they have a core set of values and beliefs
    d. all of the above are characteristics of survivors

Critical Thinking and Decision Making
1. Explain the statement, "building healthy intimate relationships and families is cyclical."
2. What are ways to improve marriages other than what the chapter lists?
3. Would you consider attending a marriage enrichment program? Why?
4. Do you tend to foresee problems before they arise or just deal with them after they happen?
5. What do you think the future of the American family will be?
6. What things should you consider before you get into a marriage enrichment program?

Answers

Key Terms: 1   myth of naturalism
              2   privatism

True/False: 1 F; 2 T; 3 T; 4 T; 5 F; 6 T; 7 F; 8 T; 9 T; 10 T

Multiple Choice: 1 c; 2 d; 3 b; 4 a; 5 b; 6 c; 7 a; 8 b; 9 c; 10 d; 11 d; 12 c; 13 b; 14 a; 15 c; 16 d; 17 b; 18 d; 19 a; 20 d; 21 c; 22 b; 23 d; 24 d; 25 d